FUNDAMENTAL GUIDE TO BECOMING THE BEST SQUASH PLAYER

FUNDAMENTAL GUIDE TO BECOMING THE BEST SQUASH PLAYER

Squash Training Course

Solly N.

FUNDAMENTAL GUIDE TO BECOMING THE BEST SQUASH PLAYER

Copyright © 2023 Solly N. All Rights Reserved.

This course contains proprietary information. No data or information of this course may be reproduced by the **[Recipient]** in any form or by any means physically, electronically including but not limited to recording, photocopying, or by any information storage and retrieval system, without permission in writing by the author.

The author retains all title, ownership, and intellectual property rights to the material and trademarks contained herein, including all supporting documentation, files, marketing material, and multimedia.

The Recipient also agrees not to duplicate or distribute or permit others to duplicate or distribute any material contained herein without the author's express written consent.

The Recipient should conduct their own due diligence investigations and an analysis of any information contained in this course and otherwise obtained before application.

The course is for information only and general in nature. It is not intended to convey any advice.

Any decisions should be taken with respect to Recipients' own individual circumstances.

All translations of this course must be approved in writing by the author. For further information to translate and seek permission for distributions and agreements, contact the author.

To order more copies individually or in bulk contact Solly N. via email sollynsquash@gmail.com.

ISBN 978-0-6457467-0-9 (Paperback)
ISBN 978-0-6457467-1-6 (E-Book)
Cover Design by nuChroma
Layout Design by nuChroma
Illustration Ideas by Solly N. (Author)
Illustration Designs by nuChroma
Vintage Image ID: JHACMK
Allam Cash Picture Library/ Alamy Stock Photo
Published by Solly N.

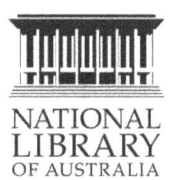

A catalogue record for this book is available from the National Library of Australia

Acknowledgment

I want to extend my sincerest gratitude and love to all the wonderful individuals who have played a role in different aspects of my life and personal growth.

First and foremost, I must express my appreciation for my mother, who is my primary motivator and holds a special place in my heart. I am also grateful to my brothers and father for their love and support in everything I do.

Additionally, I would like to express my heartfelt gratitude to my mentor Roy, who has been acting as a father figure and who has always believed in me and my vision. I am deeply grateful for his support, guidance, and help in my entrepreneurial journey, overall growth and for pushing me to reach greater heights.

Thirdly, I want to express my thanks to Erik Seversen for his mentorship and guidance for inspiring me to become an author. Thank you, Erik for helping me in getting this book finalised and published.

Furthermore, I would like to extend my gratitude to all my other mentors who have entered my life and shared their wisdom and knowledge, guiding me to become my best self.

I would also like to thank my team and club members for their unwavering support, care, and patience.

Lastly, I would like to express my gratitude to those who doubted my vision or tried to bring me down. Instead of holding grudges, I am grateful as it has pushed me to become a better person. I have learned to believe in myself, my abilities, and my vision to serve humanity globally.

Solly N.

Contents

Introduction

Welcome	01
About the Author	02
Training Planner	03
Course Study Check sheet	04

Section One
Student Briefing

Student's Code of Conduct	11
Student's Guide to Study	12

Section Two
History of Squash

Squash's Short Story	13

Section Three
V-M-G-T

Setting Vision, Mission, Goals and Targets	16

Section Four
Squash Court

Parts of the Court	20
The Two 4s	22
The Three Zones	25
Shot Types	27
Types of Balls	41

Section Five
Squash Court Rules

Scoring System	47
Decisions for Refereeing	48
How to Start the Play	48

Section Six
Fundamentals of Technique

The Grip	54
Stages of the Technique	57

Section Seven
Court Movement

Fundamentals of Movement	76
MTR-01 (Movement Training Drill)	84
MTR-02 (Movement Training Drill)	86
MTR-03 (Movement Training Drill)	88

Section Eight
Solo Training

Introduction to Solo Training	91
STR-01 (Solo Training Drill)	93
STR-02 (Solo Training Drill)	96

Section Nine
Dyads Training

Introduction to Dyads Training	99
DTR-01 (Dyads Training Drill)	100
DTR-02 (Dyads Training Drill)	102

Section Ten
Statistics- Result Tracking

What is a Statistic?	104

Section Eleven
Final Study Exercise

Key Takeaways	110

a) History of Squash
b) Squash Court
c) Squash Court Rules
d) Fundamentals of Technique
e) Court Movement
f) Solo Training Drills
g) Dyads Training Drills
h) Statistics- Result Tracking

Section Twelve
Appendix

Student's Accomplishment	114

Welcome

Welcome to the Squash Training Course **FUNDAMENTAL GUIDE TO BECOMING THE BEST SQUASH PLAYER.** This is the beginning of your squash adventure, and it consists of knowledge, ideas, practical tools, and technology to improve your squash game.

This course was designed to give you some basic tools to improve your understanding of squash and apply the information and ideas provided to accelerate your growth as a squash player.

Maximising your progress as a squash player requires a consistent and dedicated effort. By working intensively on the materials in this course, you can effectively improve your game. The key to success lies in regularly studying and applying the knowledge, ideas, practical tools, and technology covered in the course, rather than trying to absorb it all over a longer, more extended period. Consistent effort will lead to better results and a more substantial improvement in your skills on the court.

Planning is the key. It would be best for you to schedule timeslots and fill in the training planner provided on the subsequent page. The training planner can assist you in being more disciplined and keep you on track in completing this course and your on-court training.

Lastly, you need to take away the key principles from this course and apply them as much as possible to the best of your ability to make changes and improvements in your squash game. The vision is to help you become the best squash player you can be using this course.

Solly N.

About the Author

Solly N. is a visionary real estate investor, businessman, former banker, a writer, a coach, and a retired professional athlete. He is the Founder & CEO of I&B Investment Co.™.

He is also an international best-seller and co-author of PEAK PERFORMANCE: Mindset Tools for Athletes. In addition, he is a registered author with the Library of Congress and Amazon.

Since childhood, Solly was a visionary and envisioned two things:

1. To play Squash at the highest level possible and;
2. To be a successful Real Estate Investor and Businessman.

Since he arrived in Australia, he has been privileged enough to receive coaching and mentorship by some of the greatest squash players, including but not limited to:

- Former world #1- and 4-times world champion Geoff Hunt
- Former world #1 and world champion Vicki Cardwell
- Former world #5 Dan Jenson
- Former world #1 Nicol David
- Former world #3 and British Open winner Anthony Ricketts
- Former world #4 Stewart Boswell

Under their expert guidance, Solly became a world-renowned squash player. He reached the rank of #7 in the junior category and was #1 in Australia and the Oceania region.

Besides his successful squash career, Solly has devoted himself entirely to his business ventures, primarily his company I&B Investment Co.™. This Australian unlisted property fund's vision is to own entire Multi-Family Apartment (MFA) complexes, through aggregated risk that provides highly attractive rentals in safe, affordable, and healthy communities, providing both investors and tenants alike with opportunity.

His current vision is to live according to his higher consciousness and positively impact humanity globally through his experiences as a retired professional squash player and coach, his businesses, and his philanthropic endeavours.

FUNDAMENTAL GUIDE TO BECOMING THE BEST SQUASH PLAYER

Training Planner

Student's Full Name: _____

Address: _____

Mobile: _____

Email: _____

Time	Training Type	Monday	Tuesday	Wednesday	Thursday	Friday	Saturday	Sunday
06:00am								
07:00am								
08:00am								
09:00am								
10:00am								
11:00am								
12:00pm								
01:00pm								
02:00pm								
03:00pm								
04:00pm								
05:00pm								
06:00pm								
07:00pm								
08:00pm								
09:00pm								
10:00pm								

Course Study Check sheet

Student's Full Name: _____

Occupation: _____

Address: _____

Mobile: _____

Email: _____

Start Date: _____

Completed Date: _____

What is the course study check sheet?

The course study check sheet comprises all the information included in this course, including studying of sections, answering of questions and application to one's squash game at training or matches with the idea of accelerating your growth and helping you become the best squash player you can be.

How to use the course study check sheet?

This course is designed in the exact sequence so you can easily go through the entire course. Therefore, it is vital for you to go through each section one at a time without skipping to other sections.

In addition, the course also contains blank pages for answering the questions to test your understanding. It is best to follow, understand each question and write your answers as best as possible. Once each section and step is completed, turn to this check sheet and follow the below steps:

1. Put your initials on the lines;
2. Write the date completed.

The reason for initials and writing completion date is to keep you accountable and disciplined in finishing this course and to help you with your growth in your squash game.

Course timeframe:

Estimated 16 days.

Section One

Student Briefing

1.1 Study Student's Code of Conduct _____

1.2 Study Student's Guide to Study _____

Section Two

History of Squash

2.1 Study Squash's Short Story _____

2.2 Q&A Task: In your own words, describe squash

and its origins. _____

Section Three

V-M-G-T

3.1 Study Setting Vision, Mission, Goals and Targets _____

3.2 Q&A Task: Write down your V-M-G-T, then _____
pick 1 goal from each area of your goals that
you really want to achieve and describe each
one of those goals in detail. Remember, the 1
goal picked from each are the most important one from your list. To describe each of these goals, give the projected date of achievement, the colour, the type, the flavour, the smell, etc. (getting all your senses involved) of each one.

Section Four

Squash Court

4.1 Study Parts of the Court _____

4.2 Study The Two 4s _____

4.3 Study The Three Zones _____

4.4 Study Shot Types _____

4.5 Types of Balls _____

4.6 Q&A Task: Describe your understanding   _____
of the parts of the court and list all the parts
that make up a squash court?

4.7 Q&A Task: What is it meant by the below   _____
statements and in your own words, describe
the 4 Quadrants and 4 Quarters of the squash court?

"There are 4 Quadrants of the floor or surface area of the court, which is very important to understand as it helps one with the placement of the shots and movement."

"The front wall of the squash court is divided into 4 Quarters (4 Qs)."

"It was found that each four quarter of the front wall has a purpose."

4.8 Q&A Task: What is a common mistake   _____
that amateurs make when it comes to the
Three Zones?

4.9 Q&A Task: List all the basic shot types   _____
and write what their purpose is and how
can you use it?

Section Five

Squash Court Rules

5.1   Study Scoring System _____

5.2   Study Decisions for Refereeing   _____

5.3   Study How to Start the Play   _____

5.4 Q&A Task: In your own words, define the   _____
three main types of the scoring system using the
below statement as a guide:

"There are three main types of scoring system when it comes to squash games.
Hand-in-Hand-Out (HIHO) 9 points (Vintage version)
Point-A-Rally (PAR) 15 points (Older version)
Point-A-Rally (PAR) 11 points (Current version)"

5.5   Q&A Task: Write an essay describing what this statement means and give examples of Let, No Let and Stroke. You can make up a scenario or use a scenario that you have personally experienced:

"The referee then assesses the situation and will make a decision of Let, No Let or Stroke. In instances, where there are no referees present, then both the players must come to an agreement of what ruling they should accept subject to the circumstance."

5.6   Q&A Task: In your own words, define why is the statement below true?

*"It is very wise for a player to apply the principles in the preceding section **(Two 4s)** because a player can use the 4 Quarters on the front wall and the 4 Quadrants to strategically construct and win rallies."*

Section Six

Fundamentals of Technique

6.1   Study The Grip

6.2   Study Stages of the Technique

6.3   Q&A Task: In your own words, write down all the steps of Handshake or V Shape grip to test your understanding? Also, define why the is the statement below true?

"The squash racket grip is one of the most basic, important, and neglected parts of a squash technique whether it's on the forehand (FH) or backhand (BH)."

6.4   Q&A Task: In your own words, define why the statement below is true and write down all the steps of the three stages of the technique?

"Preparation of the racket from the "T" is one of the most crucial parts in striking a clean ball. Without solid preparation, one cannot move and strike a clean ball because one won't have the time due to the racket not being prepared and in the right position."

6.5   Q&A Task: In your own words, write down all the steps of the forehand (FH) technique?

6.6 Q&A Task: In your own words, write down _____
all the steps of the backhand (BH) technique?

Section Seven

Court Movement

7.1 Study Fundamentals of Movement _____

7.2 Practical: MTR-01 (Movement Training Drill) _____

7.3 Q&A Task: Describe any wins or results _____
you have gained from applying the MTR-01?

7.3 Practical: MTR-02 (Movement Training Drill) _____

7.4 Q&A Task: Describe any wins or results _____
you have gained from applying the MTR-02?

7.5 Practical: MTR-03 (Movement Training Drill) _____

7.6 Q&A Task: Describe any wins or results _____
you have gained from applying the MTR-03?

Section Eight

Solo Training

8.1 Study Introduction to Solo Training _____

8.2 Practical: STR-01 (Solo Training Drill) _____

8.3 Q&A Task: Describe any wins or results _____
you have gained from applying the STR-01?

8.4 Practical: STR-02 (Solo Training Drill) _____

8.5 Q&A Task: Describe any wins or results _____
you have gained from applying the STR-02?

Section Nine

Dyads Training

9.1 Study Introduction to Dyads Training _____

9.2 **Practical:** DTR-01 (Dyads Training Drill) _____

9.3 **Q&A Task:** Describe any wins or results that _____
you have gained from applying the DTR-01?

9.4 **Practical:** DTR-02 (Dyads Training Drill) _____

9.5 **Q&A Task:** Describe any wins or results that _____
you have gained from applying the DTR-02?

Section Ten

Statistics- Result Tracking

10.1 Study What is a Statistic? _____

10.2 **Q&A Task:** Describe in your own words,
your understanding of the below statement
and draw a rough sketch of an up, down
and stable statistics?

"Statistics are simple, they can be understood as:

An up statistic means that the current amount or number is more than the preceding one.

A down statistic means that the current amount or number is less than the preceding one.

A stable statistic means that the current amount or number is close or identical to the preceding without any improvement or deterioration."

Section Eleven

Final Study Exercise

11.1 Q&A Task: Write about what you have learnt from this course, the key takeaways, and how can you apply the information to help you become the best squash player you can be? Go through each item below.

      a)   History of Squash
      b)   Squash Court
      c)   Squash Court Rules
      d)   Fundamentals of Technique
      e)   Court Movement
      f)   Solo Training Drills
      g)   Group Training Drills
      h)   Statistics- Result Tracking _____

Section Twelve

Appendix

12.1 Q&A Task: Student's Accomplishment _____

Section One

Student Briefing

1.1 Student's Code of Conduct

The Student's Code of Conduct is a behavioural guide for this course to get you through the study materials and the course successfully and with ease. Therefore, some rules and guidelines must be followed to bring the best result possible for you. They are as follows:

1) Be punctual with your time when studying and doing practical tasks.

2) Always use your Training Planner in the preceding section of this course as a guide.

3) Do not take drugs or alcohol when studying this course or on practical tasks. Prescriptive drugs from a health practitioner are an exception.

4) Do not take alcohol within 24-48 hours when working on this course or practical tasks.

5) Start your day by drinking 600ml to 1 litre of water first thing in the morning and staying hydrated throughout the day.

6) Be disciplined with good and healthy consumption of food.

7) Get at least 7-8 hours of sleep when studying this course or practical tasks.

8) Avoid any distractions, whether phone or other communication devices, whilst studying the course and practical tasks.

9) If you don't understand or require further assistance with anything related to this course, then contact Solly via email sollynsquash@gmail.com.

1.2 Student's Guide to Study

The author believes that understanding vocabulary is key to effectively learning any subject. When studying this course, it is important to fully comprehend all the information presented. Do not skip over any words or phrases that are unclear. Instead, take the time to look up their meaning and context to ensure a complete understanding. Using a dictionary can help understand a word's meaning in a particular context. Avoid assumptions, as they can lead to confusion. To maximise your learning experience and minimise confusion, make sure to clarify every difficult word.

Section Two

History of Squash

2.1 Squash's Short Story

Squash is a world-renowned sport, and its history is filled with great and inspiring stories throughout the years. In its early days, the game of squash was played in different locations from eminent private schools and universities, consisting of exclusive private men's clubs. The game was also played on famous ships.

You may ask what is squash and what are its origins?

Squash is a racket sport which requires an incredible amount of hand-and-eye coordination played as an individual or by two or four players in a four-walled court with a rubber ball. The game's objective is to hit the ball in such a way that the ball makes the front wall and in the parts of the court where another player cannot retrieve the ball on the first bounce.

Squash originated from the game of rackets and was first played in London prisons in the 19th century. However, it was at Harrow School in the 1830s where students discovered the exciting potential of the game. They noticed that a punctured ball that squished upon impact with the wall made for a more thrilling game. Quickly, the game spread to other schools. Initially, the courts at Harrow were hazardous due to their proximity to pipes, water, cliffs, and other obstacles. The students soon realised natural rubber was the best material for the squash ball. They also modified their rackets for a smaller reach and improved playability in tight conditions. By 1864, the school had constructed four outdoor courts for the game.

During the 20th century, squash's popularity increased across various clubs, schools and private individuals who built squash courts without any dimensions.

In 1884 North America, the first squash court was at St. Paul's School in Concord, New Hampshire.

In 1904 Philadelphia, Pennsylvania, the United States Squash Rackets Association was formed, now known as the U.S. Squash.

In 1907, a subcommittee called the Tennis, Rackets & Fives Association of Queens, New York was formed to set standards for squash which regulated the three sports (Fives being a similar sport that uses hands instead of rackets).

In 1912, the subcommittee published the rules of squash, which combined aspects of three sports. In addition, the RMS Titanic had a squash court for the first class. On the G-Deck, the 1st-Class squash court was situated with the spectators viewing gallery being one level higher on F-Deck. The passengers on RMS Titanic were allowed to use the court for one hour unless other passengers were waiting.

In 1923, the Royal Automobile Club hosted a meeting to discuss squash rules and regulations further. After five years, to set standards for the game in Great Britain and internationally, the Squash Rackets Association, now known as England Squash, was formed. The rackets at the time were formed from a piece of English ash, with a suede (leather with a napped surface), leather grip and natural gut.

Squash spread globally by the 1950s, leading to the emergence of Hashim Khan on the squash scene. Born in a small village near Peshawar, Pakistan, Hashim began his career as a ball boy at a local British Officer's Club. As he honed his skills, he became a local squash professional. In 1951, he won the British Open tournament (the Wimbledon of squash) with ease.

Over the years, squash has grown into a prominent sport worldwide, evolving continuously. It has produced some of the world's best players, including legends such as Heather Mackay, Jonah Barrington, Geoff Hunt, Jahangir Khan, Jansher Khan, and more, who have made significant contributions to the sport.

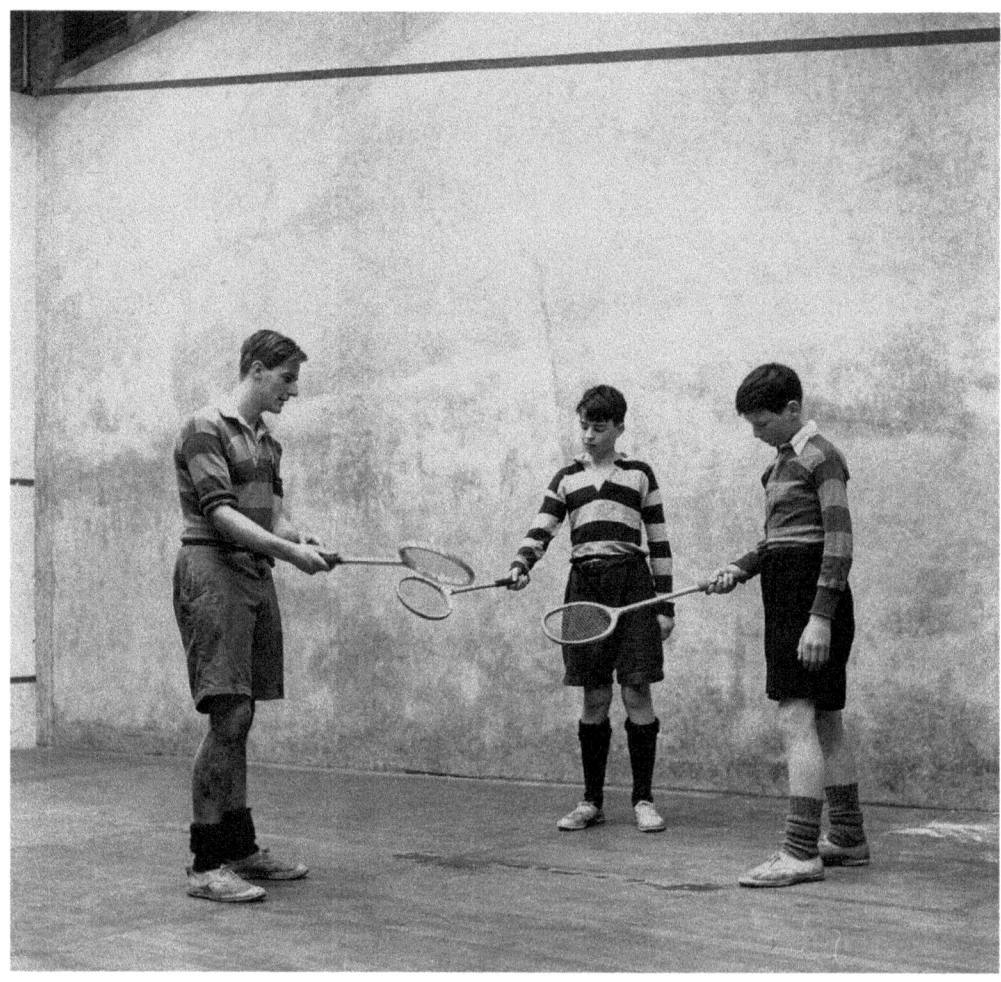

Learning the art of Squash at Haileybury College in 1948

Full Name: _____

Date: _____

2.2 **Q&A Task:** In your own words, describe squash and its origins.

_____

_____

_____

_____

_____

_____

_____

_____

_____

_____

_____

_____

_____

_____

_____

_____

_____

_____

_____

Section Three

V-M-G-T

3.1 Setting Vision, Mission, Goals and Targets

The author believes that drive, determination, and big thinking are crucial for success, but even more important is clarity on one's vision, mission, goals, and targets, also known as V-M-G-T. In this section, the author explains the meaning of V-M-G-T and why it's crucial to set them. Setting V-M-G-T not only brings clarity but also shapes one's self-image and future aspirations.

The author has discovered through research and experience that understanding V-M-G-T and building a strong self-image can help achieve great things, such as healing illness, becoming a top athlete, or building successful businesses. So, how does one define Vision, Mission, Goals, and Targets?

- **Vision** is a big, imagined objective that guides one's actions. It's often on a global or universal scale.
- **Mission** is the reason behind the vision.
- **Goal** is a long-term objective that takes a year or more to achieve.
- **Target** is an objective or result towards which efforts are directed. It is a specific, actionable task aligned with vision, mission, and goal, with specific milestones that can be hourly, daily, weekly, monthly, quarterly etc.

It's crucial that V-M-G-T are aligned, as misalignment leads to confusion and incomplete or no achievement of V-M-G-T. Think of a sailboat and its sailors. The sailors have a vision of sailing from one continent to another, the mission is why they want to make the journey, the goal is the compass that helps with the direction, planning, and timeline, and the target is the actionable steps taken along the way, like hourly, daily, weekly, monthly tasks.

Once the meaning of V-M-G-T is clear, the next step is to build one's self-image. The author has created an exercise for this, which can be applied in personal or athletic pursuits, not just in squash. The exercise involves sitting in a quiet room with a blank piece of paper and contemplating questions such as:

1) What is one's vision and mission in life or for the sport of squash?
2) What are one's goals and targets to help one achieve their vision and mission in life or for the sport of squash?
3) What value can one add to his family, community, country, and the world in life or through the sport of squash?
4) What does one need to do to achieve his V-M-G-T in life or for the sport of squash?

When performing the above exercise, one needs to follow the below steps to achieve optimum results:

1) Write V-M-G-T to cover all areas of your life (beyond just sport squash), such as self-betterment, health, relationships, finance, work, business, and community
2) Make V-M-G-T as big as you want and think big
3) Respond to the above questions by writing it in the present tense and in detail
4) Be crystal clear with everything that you are writing as it plays a major role in achieving the V-M-G-T
5) Write down the date on which you want to achieve the V-M-G-T
6) Write "thank you, thank you, thank you" and the current day's date on the paper
7) Bring your spirit, mind, and body in line and visualise your V-M-G-T
8) Expect and feel it strongly that you have already attracted the desired V-M-G-T
9) Believe that by writing it down, the manifestation of the desired has started

Now for the third and final aspect of becoming and attracting the success you desire in your life—you must commit to your vision and mission and take daily actions. The reason being, without commitment and daily actions, you are not doing your part.

Full Name: _____

Date: _____

3.2   Q&A Task: Write down your V-M-G-T then pick 1 goal from each area of your goals that you really want to achieve and describe each one of those goals in detail? Remember, the 1 goal picked from each area is the most important on your list. To describe each of these 1 goals from each area, give the projected date of achievement, the colour, the type, the flavour, the smell, etc. (getting all your senses involved) for each one.

_____

_____

_____

_____

_____

_____

_____

_____

_____

_____

_____

_____

Section Four

Squash Court

4.1 Parts of the Court

The playing area of a squash court is surrounded by four walls and has a solid beech floor that provides a springy surface for player comfort and reduces leg strain. The court is marked with various lines, including two service boxes, a tin, "T" position, outline, service line, short or front line, and a half court line, which are used to set rules for play. *(Refer to Illustration 1: Parts of the court)*

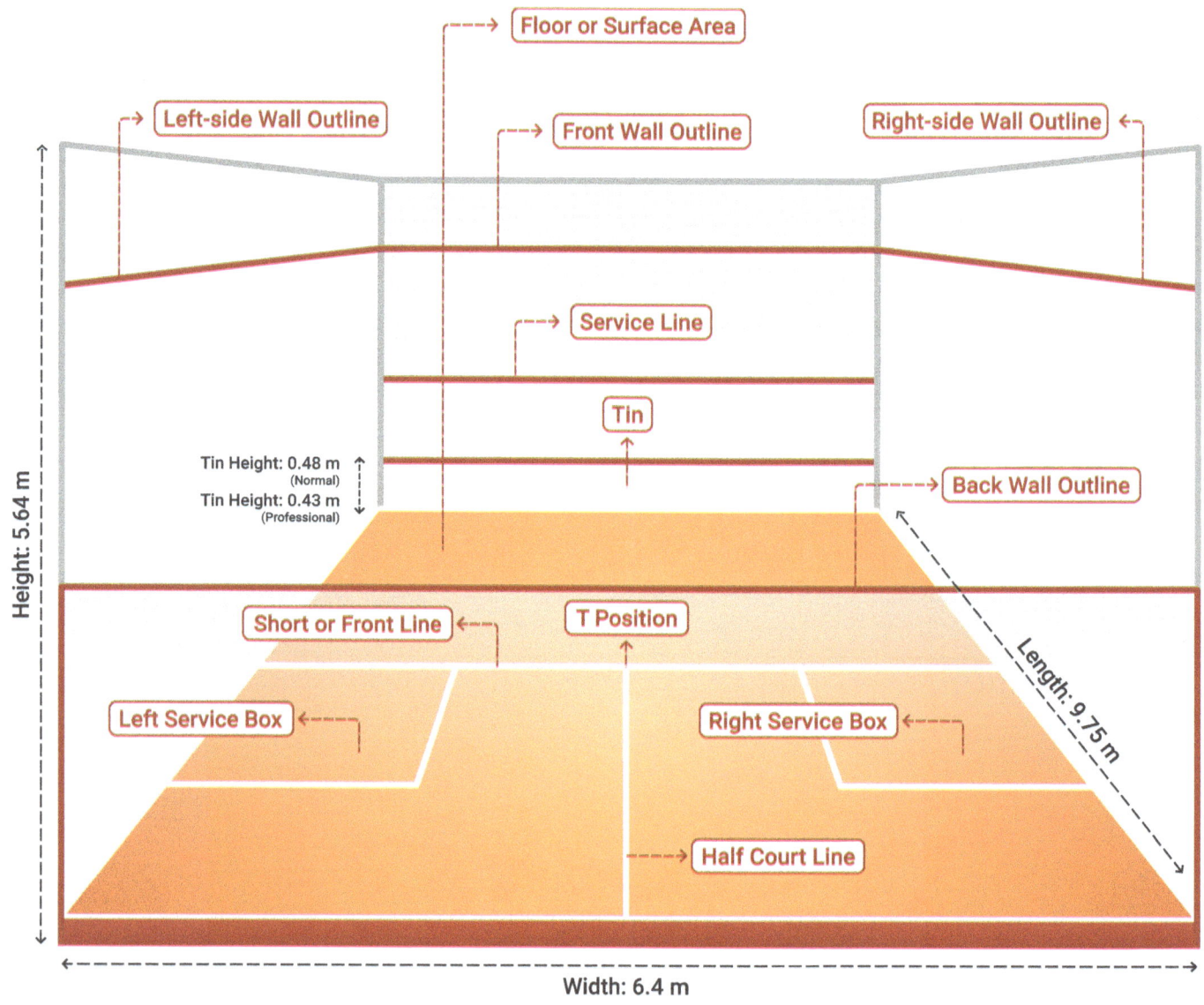

Illustration 1: Parts of the Court

Four Walls:

The four walls are divided into a front wall, two side walls, and a back wall. There are different types of materials that can be used to build the four walls of a squash court. These can be fabricated panel walls, plastered walls, high density boards, sand-filled system walls and glass walls.

Floor or Surface:

The court's surface is made of a solid beech floor which provides a spring for players comfort which reduces leg strain.

Service Boxes:

The back two boxes (back right box and back left box) contain smaller boxes called service boxes.

Tin:

The bottom of the front wall of the squash court is called a tin. A tin is a half meter-high metal area with a line on top of it.

"T" Position:

"T" position is situated in the middle part of the court where the short or front line is. It is the central position of the court. The player who controls the "T" position is in control of the game.

Outline:

An outline runs along the top of the front wall which descends along both the side walls and to the back wall.

Service Line:

The service line is a middle line situated on the front wall.

Short or Front Line:

A court's floor or surface consists of a short or front line that separates the front and back of the court.

Half Court Line:

The half court line separates the right and left sides of the back portion of the court. This results in the creation of three boxes.

The dimensions of a singles squash court in metres (m) are as follows:

Length of a squash court is 9.75m
Width of a squash court is 6.4m
Height of a squash court is 5.64m
Tin height of a squash court is 0.48m for normal play and 0.43m for professionals.

4.2 The Two 4s

The Two 4s are separated into two parts:

1) The Front wall of the court is broken into 4 Quarters and;
2) The Floor or Surface area of the court is broken into 4 Quadrants.

The Two 4s were designed to simplify the placement of the ball on a squash court. The ball hitting at a specific part of the front wall is what we call the 'cause' and the ball falling at a particular target on the floor or surface area of the court is called an 'effect'. Therefore, it was discovered that if a player were to hit a particular quarter of the front wall, then the ball would end up in a particular area of the floor or surface area. The Two 4s are vital to a player's learning as it helps one break the court and simplify the target hitting on a squash court.

4 Quadrants of the Floor or Surface:

There are 4 Quadrants of the floor or surface area of the court which is very important to understand as it helps one with the placement of the shots as well as movement. To put this into perspective, let's imagine the floor or surface area of the court, and we will divide that into what we call our 4 Quadrants. To do that, we will draw a line from the T area where the short or front line is located and draw a straight line all the way to the front wall where the tin is. This helps us break the court into 4 Quadrants.

Quadrant 1 is located on the front left-hand corner, also known as the front backhand (BH) corner.

Quadrant 2 is located on the front right-hand corner, also known as the front forehand (FH) corner.

Quadrant 3 is situated on the back left-hand corner, commonly known as the back backhand (BH) corner.

Quadrant 4 is situated on the back right-hand corner, also called the back forehand (FH) corner.

In addition, within each 4 Quadrants, there are 4 small pies, with one pie located in each corner of the 4 quadrants. The pies play a vital part because this is where a ball should ideally end up when practising or playing. *(Refer to Illustration 2: 4 Quadrants)*

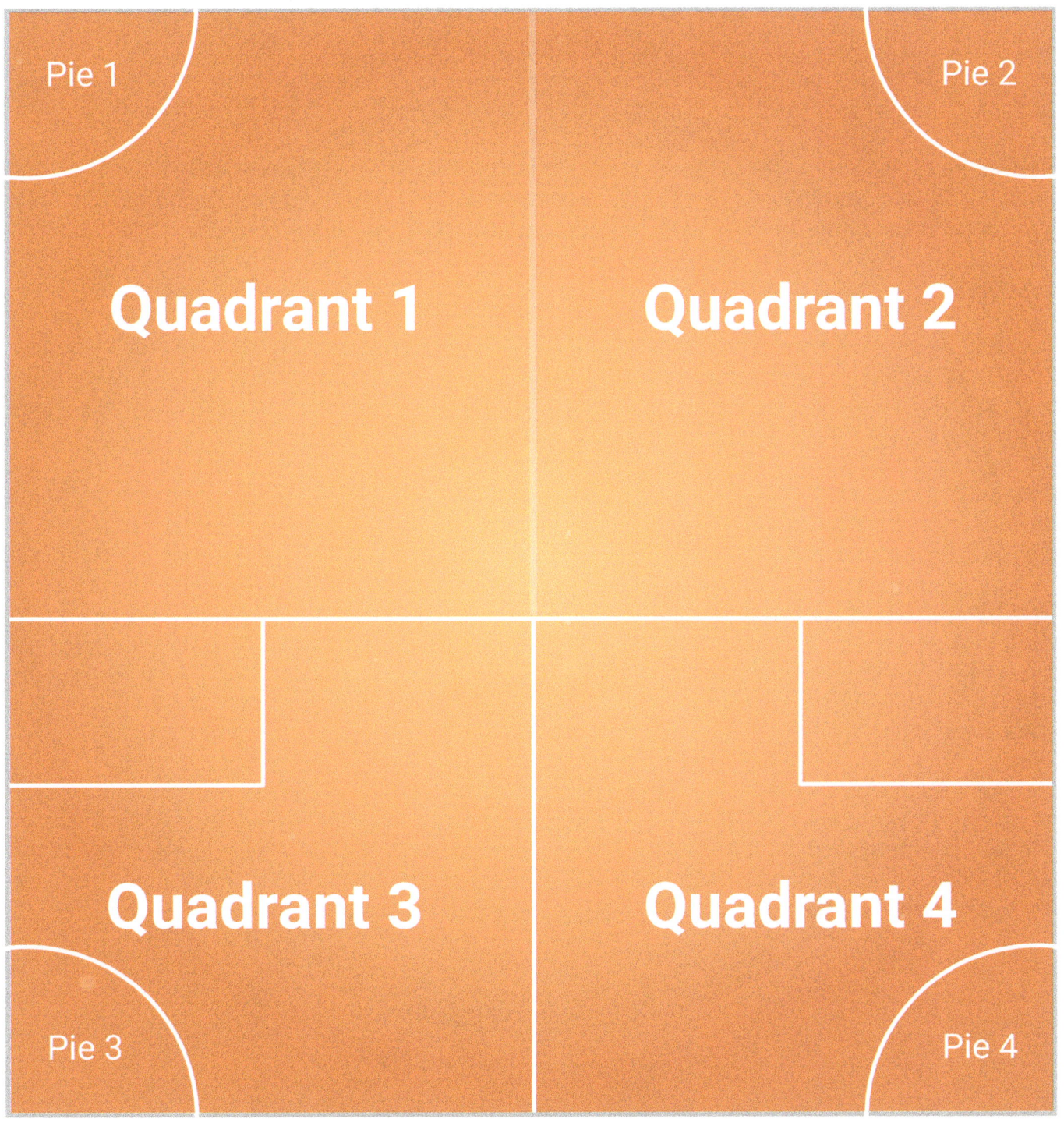

Illustration 2: 4 Quadrants

4 Quarters or 4 Qs of the Front Wall:

The front wall of the squash court is divided into 4 Quarters (4 Qs). We will start from the bottom of the front wall and work all the way to the top finishing at the outline of the front wall.

Imagine a line drawn between the tin and the service line. We will call the bottom one just above the tin our First Quarter (Q1), whilst the one below the service line and First Quarter is called Second Quarter (Q2).

We will then take the front wall starting from the service line to the outline of the front line and draw a line between the two, and break it into two more quarters. Thus, giving us our Third quarter (Q3) above the service line and Fourth quarter (Q4) under the outline.

Each of the four quarters of the front wall in a squash court serves a specific purpose.

Quarter 1 is used for short shots that bounce in either the front backhand or front forehand area. These can include straight drop shots, cross drop shots, cross court kills, straight kills, trickle boasts, Aussie boasts, cross court nicks of the bounce, cross court nicks of the volley, or straight volley drops from both the backhand and forehand.

Quarter 2 is used for shots that are hit from the front of the court to the back, either as a straight drive or cross court drive from the forehand or backhand. The intention is to get the ball to bounce first past the service box area and then into the back part of the court, also known as the "pie".

Quarter 3 is a crucial quarter for hitting straight or cross court volley drives from the T and short line. The intention is to get the ball to the back of the court, with the first bounce behind the service box area and the second bounce into the "pie". This quarter can also be used for straight drives or cross court drives from the back part of the court. The back part of the court is considered a key area in constructing rallies.

Quarter 4 is the top of the front wall and is used to buy time under pressure. High shots such as straight lobs, cross lobs, or even corkscrew shots from the backhand or forehand can be used in this area. This quarter can be utilised from both the front and back areas of the court. (Disclaimer: Corkscrews are used as an attacking shot and not under pressure as it requires angle and good positioning). *(Refer to Illustration 3: 4 Quarters or 4 Qs)*

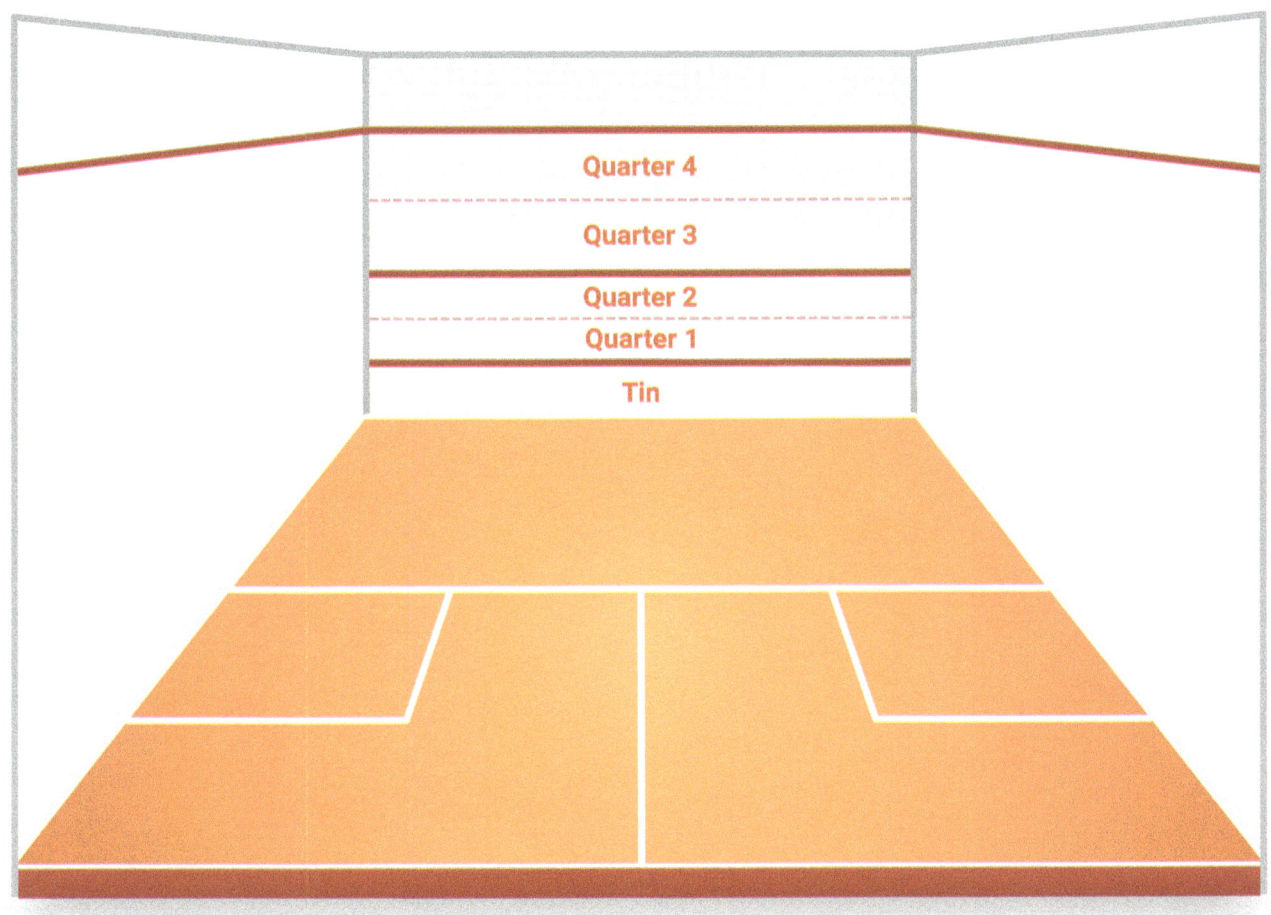

Illustration 3: 4 Quarters or 4 Qs

4.3 The Three Zones

The common mistake that a lot of amateur players make, especially when they are on the T or the short line is to take the ball late which means that the players tend to take or play the ball behind themselves either inside Quadrant 3 or Quadrant 4, often due to waiting for the ball. This results in the ball going past them and dying at the back part of the court. To solve that problem, the Three Zones were created.

To explain what the Three Zones are, we will take as an example of Quadrant 4 on the floor or surface area of the court which is situated at the back forehand corner of the court. We will then break Quadrant 4 into 3 quarters, drawing one line from the service box to the half court line to make it our Zone 1, then another line between Zone 1 and the back wall, which will divide it into Zone 2 and Zone 3.

When playing straight drives or cross court drives to the back of the court, it is essential that a ball must be played either on the first bounce or volleying it (playing it on the full or the ball up in the air not yet bounced) when in Zone 1 and Zone 2. This will result in helping a player take the ball early and save the ball from going past or worse dying in the back corner or in the pie. A ball can be played on the first bounce as it bounces in Zone 3 because it will often bounce off the back wall. It is prudent to always play the ball within Zone 1 and Zone 2. **(Refer to Illustration 4: The Three Zones)**

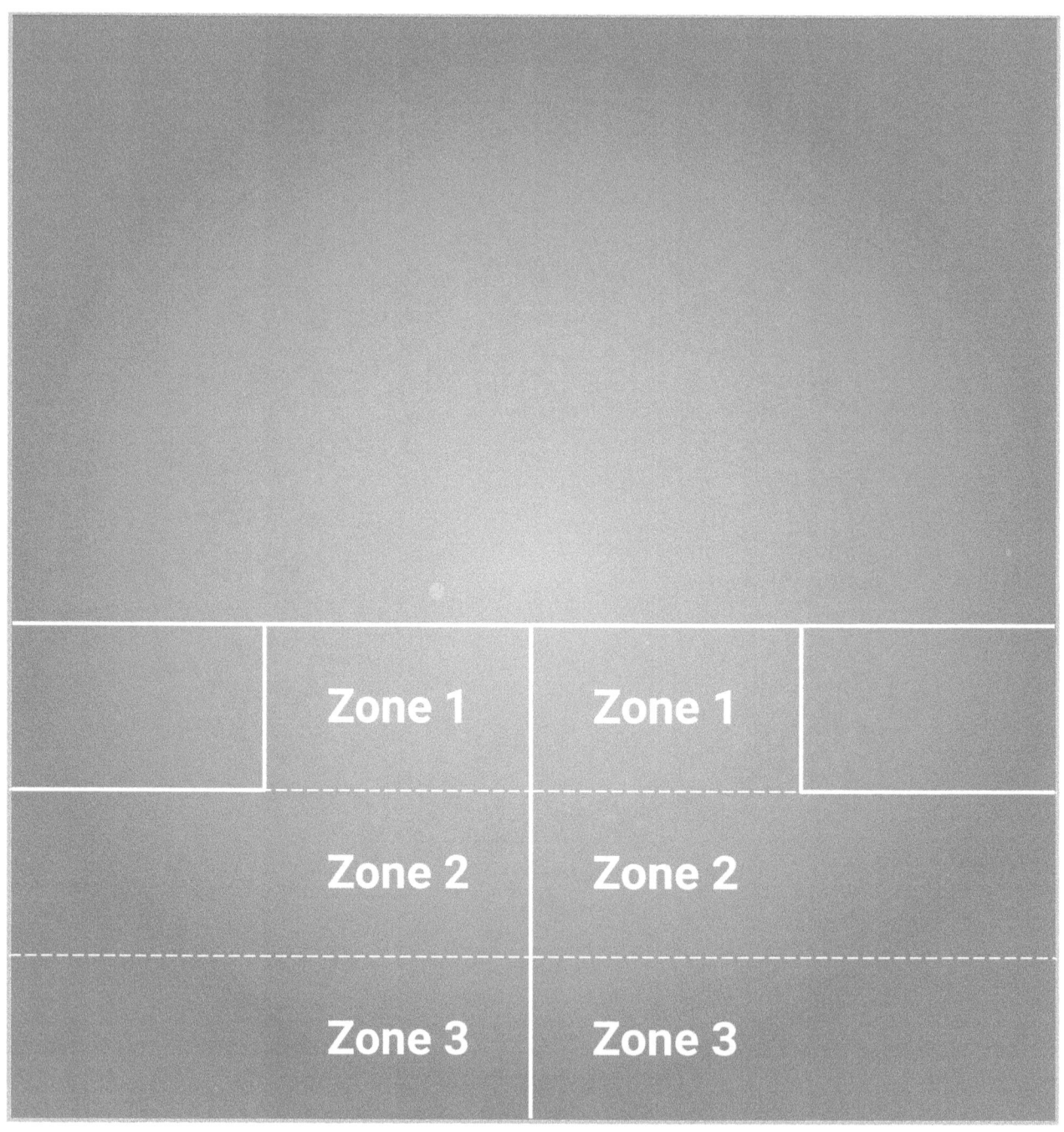

Illustration 4: The Three Zones

4.4 Shot Types

Knowing the different shot types and understanding what they are, and what they mean is crucial to one's growth as a squash player. The most elite professional squash players worldwide first look to master the basic shots of the game before adding other fancy shot types. In this section, we will cover the basic shot types and their meaning. Carefully study this section because this can assist you in understanding the game further.

Straight Drive:

Straight drive, also known as a straight length, is one of the fundamental and most played shots in a squash game as it is the base of the game, and it helps one construct the base and the rallies. The straight drive is played either on the forehand or backhand. The purpose of hitting a straight drive is to play as tight along the side wall so it makes it difficult for one to retrieve.

The straight drive is a shot played with medium or hard paced that is hit on the front wall on Quarter 2 and 3, which gets the ball into the back corner behind the service box or Zone 2 with the second bounce dying in Zone 3 or the pie. Played right and tight on the side wall, either on the forehand or backhand, it can not only win rallies but it also helps take the opponent away from the "T" position or central part of the court. *(Refer to Illustration 5: Shot Type - Straight Drive BH and Illustration 6: Shot Type - Straight Drive FH)*

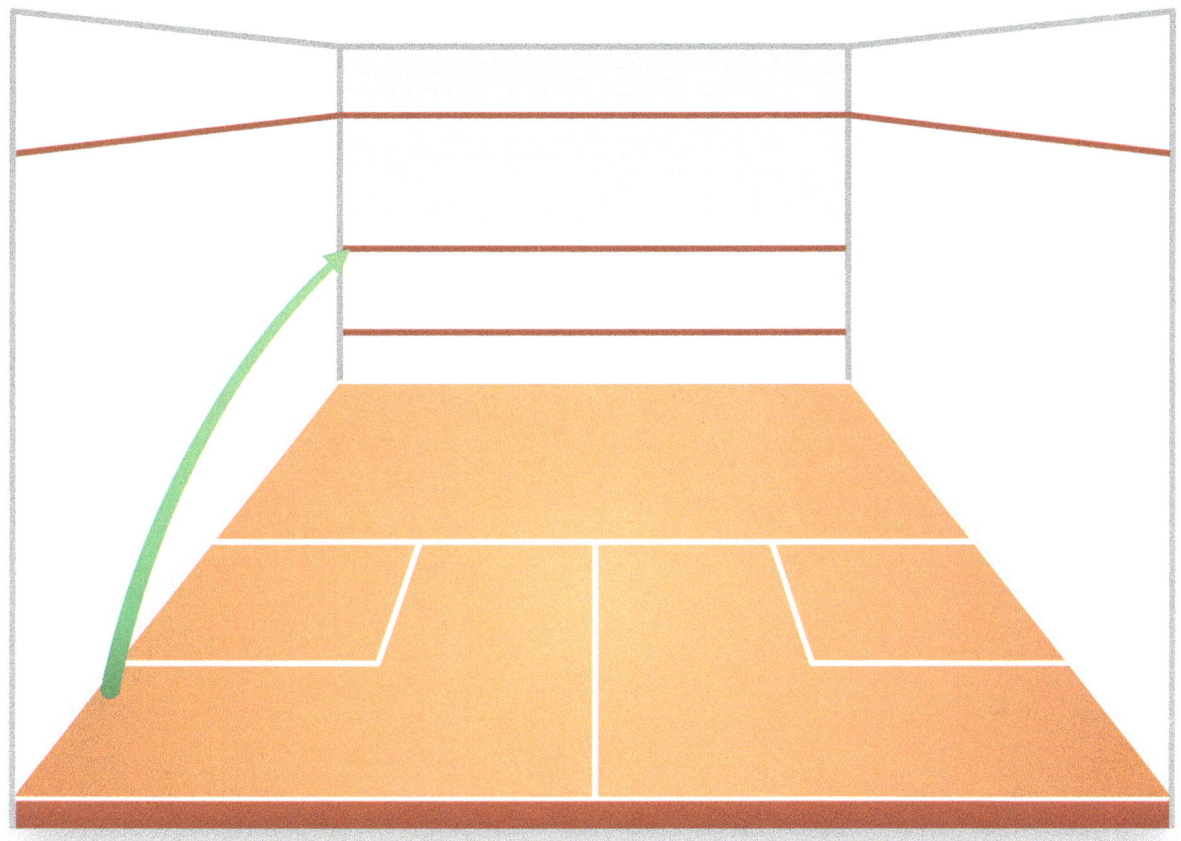

Illustration 5: Shot Type - Straight Drive BH

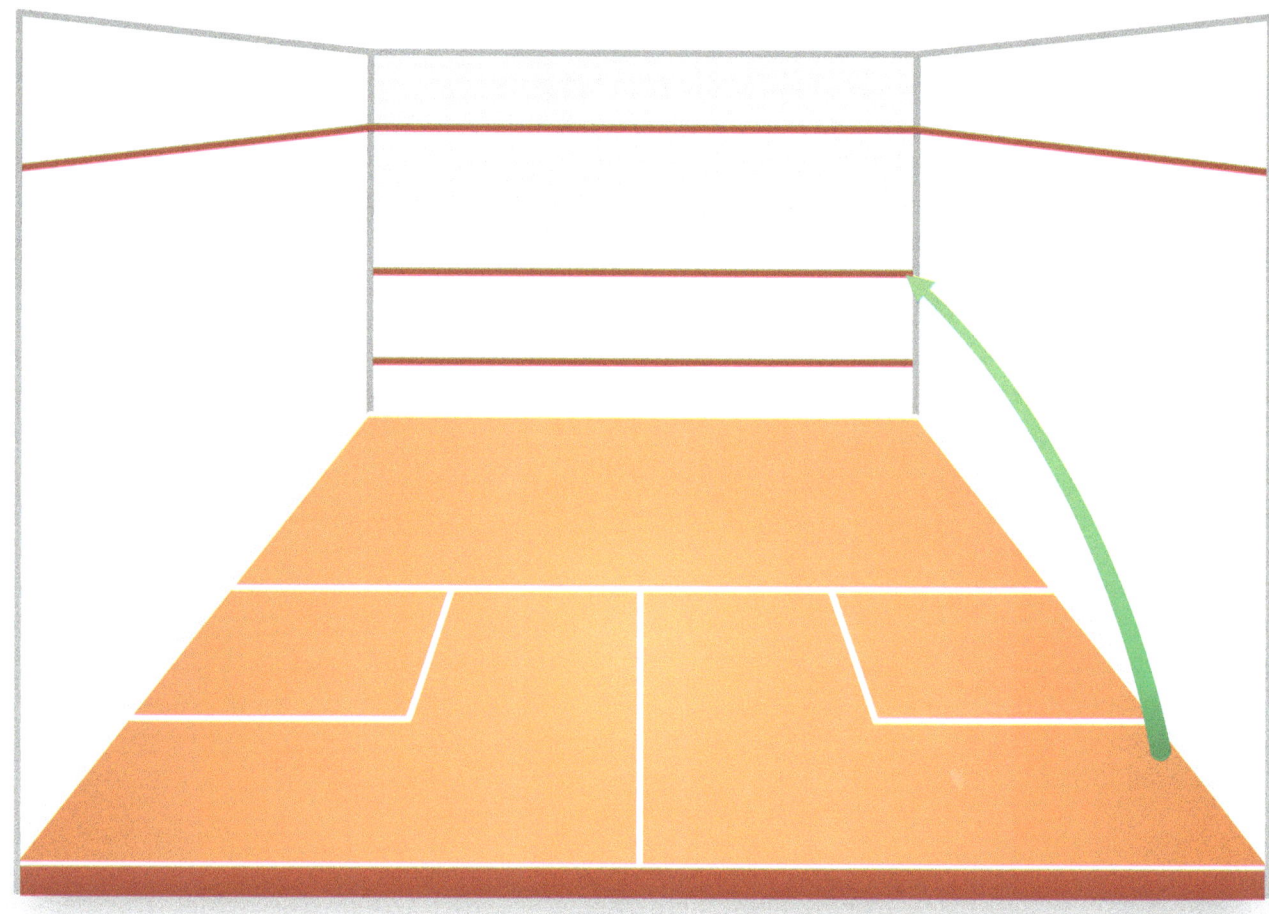

Illustration 6: Shot Type - Straight Drive FH

Cross-court Drive:

Cross-court drive or cross court length is another fundamental and most played shot in the game. The cross-court drive is like a straight drive which can be played as a forehand or backhand. The purpose of hitting a cross court drive is to switch the sides or Quadrants in which the game is played. The cross-court drive is a shot played with medium or hard paced that is hit on the middle of the front wall on Quarter 2 and 3 which gets the ball into the back corner behind the service box or Zone 2 with second bounce dying in Zone 3 or the pie. Played right and with an angle, one can win outright rallies by hitting a nick. (Nick is the part of the sidewalls which meets the floor and when a ball hits in that area, it causes an outright winner). It is one of the best shots to take the opponent away from the "T" position or central part of the court. *(Refer to Illustration 7: Shot Type - Cross-court Drive BH and Illustration 8: Shot Type - Cross-court Drive FH)*

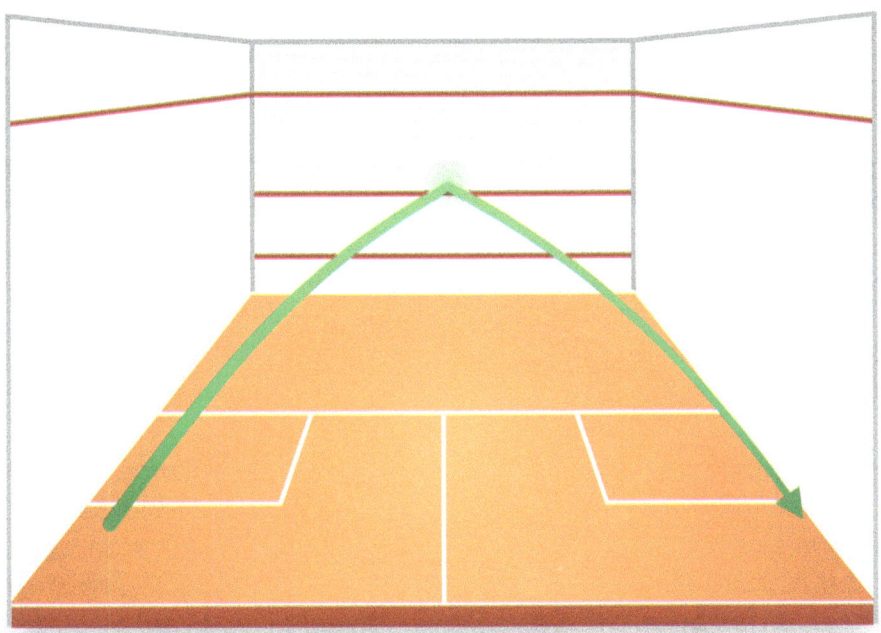

Illustration 7: Shot Type - Cross-court Drive BH

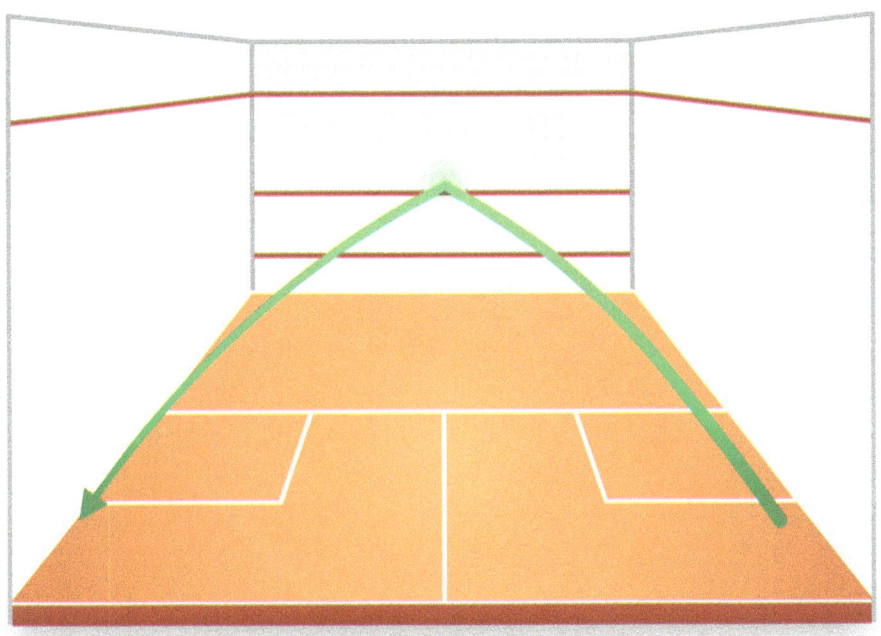

Illustration 8: Shot Type - Cross-court Drive FH

Boast:

Boasts are effective shots for both attacking and defending in squash. When used as an attacking shot, the aim is to move the player away from the "T". When used as a defensive shot, it helps a player escape a tight situation, such as when they are at a full stretch in the back corner.

There are two types of boasts: two-wall and three-wall. Both are played to create angles and can be used for attacking or defensive purposes, with the latter being more commonly used as a defensive shot.

A two-wall boast is executed by hitting the side wall at an angle, followed by hitting the middle of the front wall in Quarter 1. The ball should bounce twice or three times before reaching the side wall. This is an attacking boast that can be played with a soft, medium, or hard pace.

A three-wall boast involves hitting the side wall at an angle, followed by hitting the front wall in Quarter 1, and then the side wall. It can be played with soft, medium, or hard pace as an attacking shot, with the goal of hitting the nick. As a defensive shot, the same steps are followed, but the ball is aimed higher, typically at Quarter 2 or 3. **(Refer to Illustration 9: Shot Type - Boast (Two Wall) FH, Illustration 10: Shot Type - Boast (Two Wall) BH, Illustration 11: Shot Type - Boast (Three Wall) FH and Illustration 12: Shot Type - Boast (Three Wall) BH)**

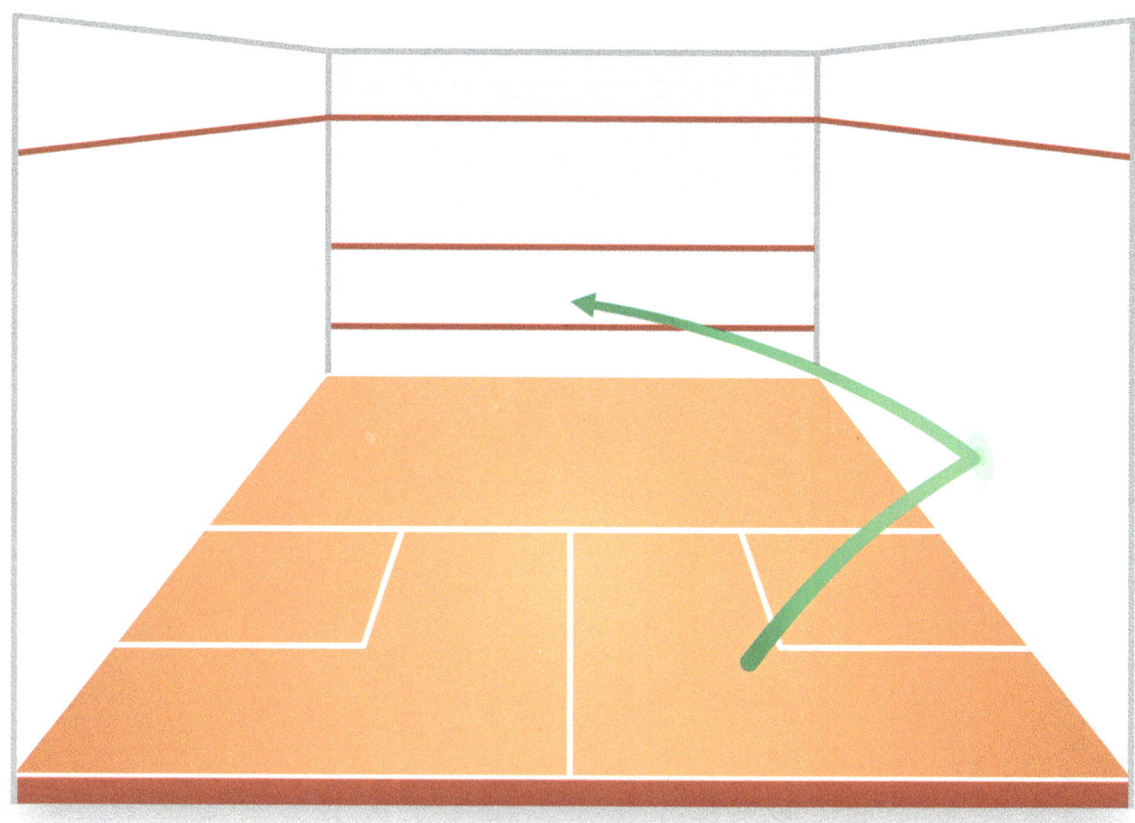

Illustration 9: Shot Type - Boast (Two Wall) FH

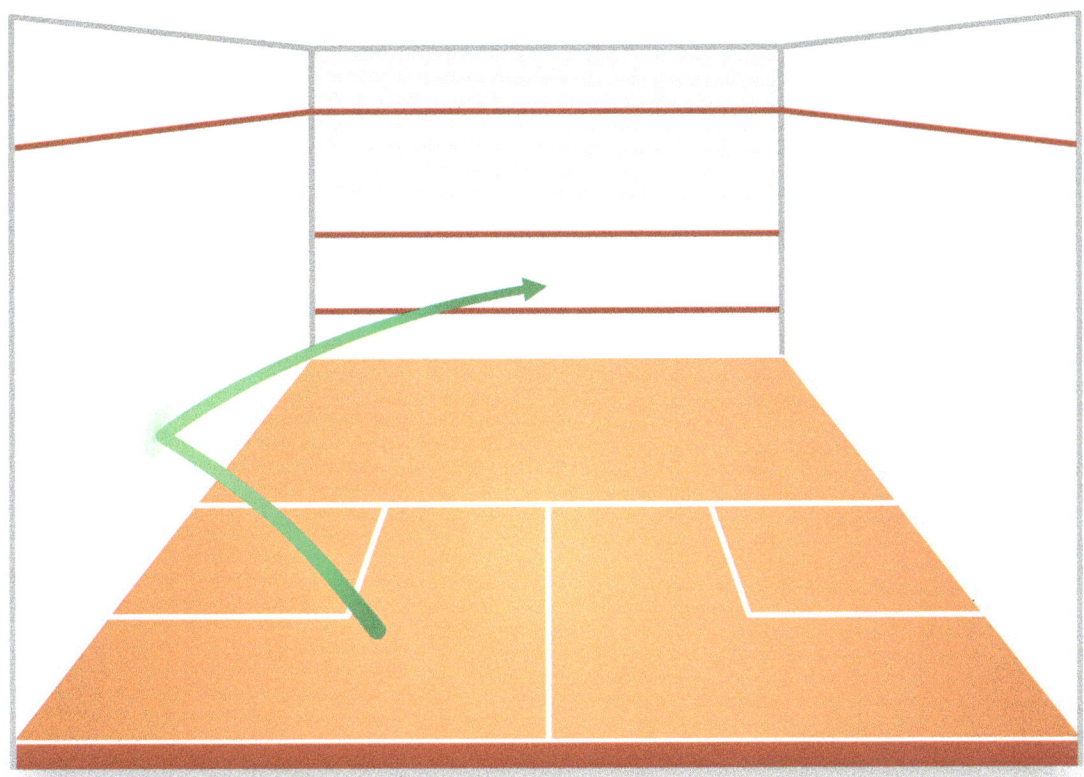

Illustration 10: Shot Type - Boast (Two Wall) BH

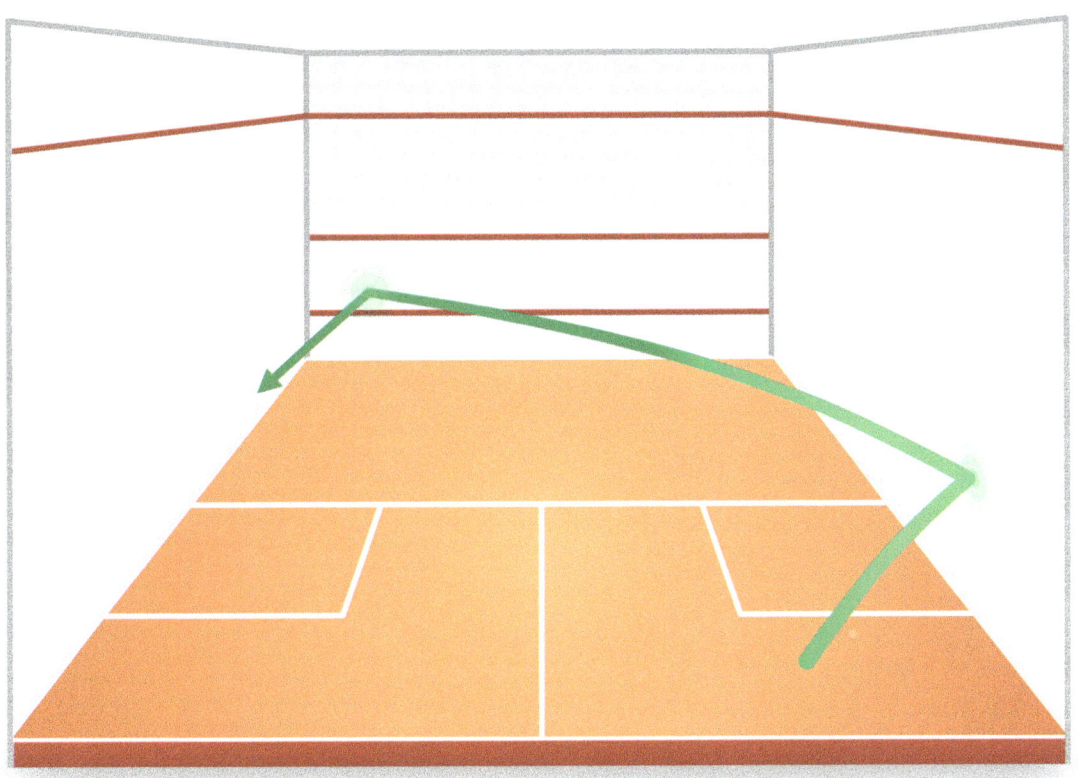

Illustration 11: Shot Type - Boast (Three Wall) FH

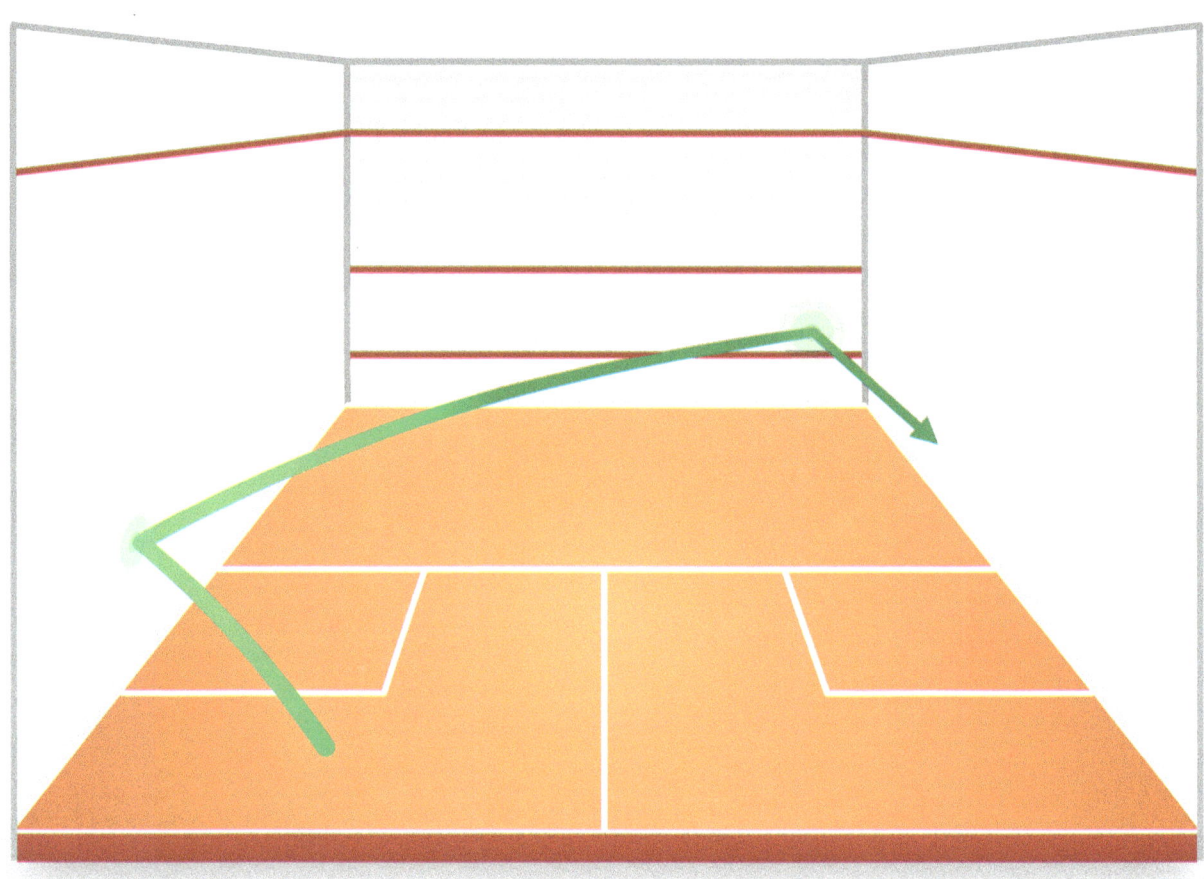

Illustration 12: Shot Type - Boast (Three Wall) BH

Volley:

The volley is an important and often underutilised shot by amateurs. It's a shot played before the ball touches the ground, playing it on the full or when it is still in the air. Volleys are usually executed as an attacking shot and allows one to control the "T" and short line. The player who can execute volleys effectively usually controls the "T" and the game.

Volleys are typically aimed at the front wall and are played in Quarters 1, 3, and 4, depending on the type of volley used. To target Quarters 3 and 4, the ball should be hit straight or cross court in those quarters. The intent is to have the ball's second bounce occur inside Zone 3 or the back corners.

In Quarter 1, volleys can also be used for short attacks, such as straight volley drops (hard or soft), cross volleys (hard or soft), volley boasts (hard or soft), and cross court nicks (hard or soft). ***(Refer to Illustration 13: Shot Type - Volley BH and Illustration 14: Shot Type - Volley FH)***

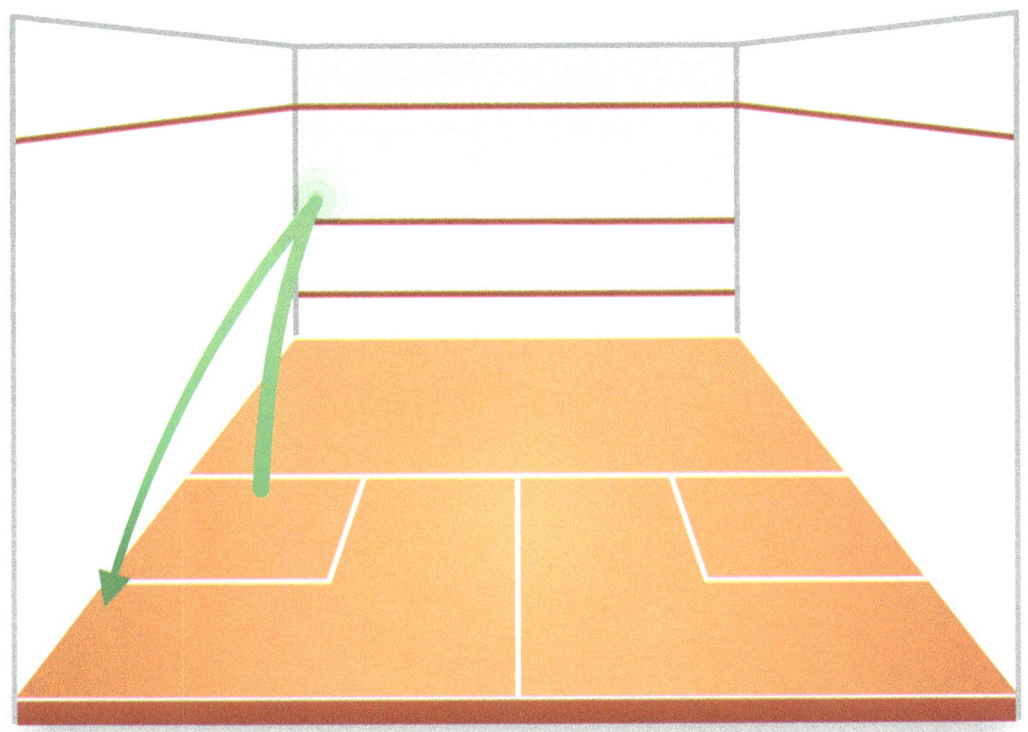

Illustration 13: Shot Type - Volley BH

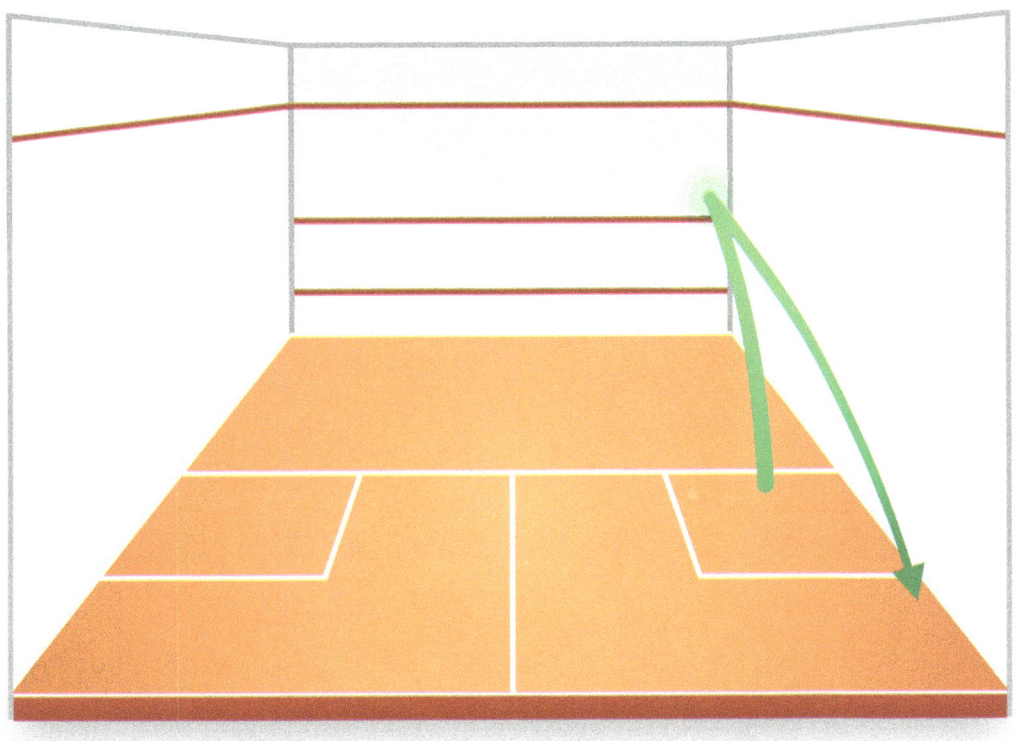

Illustration 14: Shot Type - Volley FH

Drop:

Drop is a critical shot in the game as it is the opposite of straight or crosscourt drives. The purpose of the shot is to move the player to the front part of the court away from the "T". It is typically played nice and softly in a way on the front wall in Quarter 1 so the ball drops and stays short in the front corners or inside the pie. A drop shot can be played straight, making it tight and stick to the side wall or played, so it catches the nick. A drop shot can also be played as a cross drop, hitting in the middle of Quarter 1 on the front wall with the aim of it bouncing more than twice before an opponent reaches for it. ***(Refer to Illustration 15: Shot Type - Drop FH and Illustration 16: Shot Type - Drop BH)***

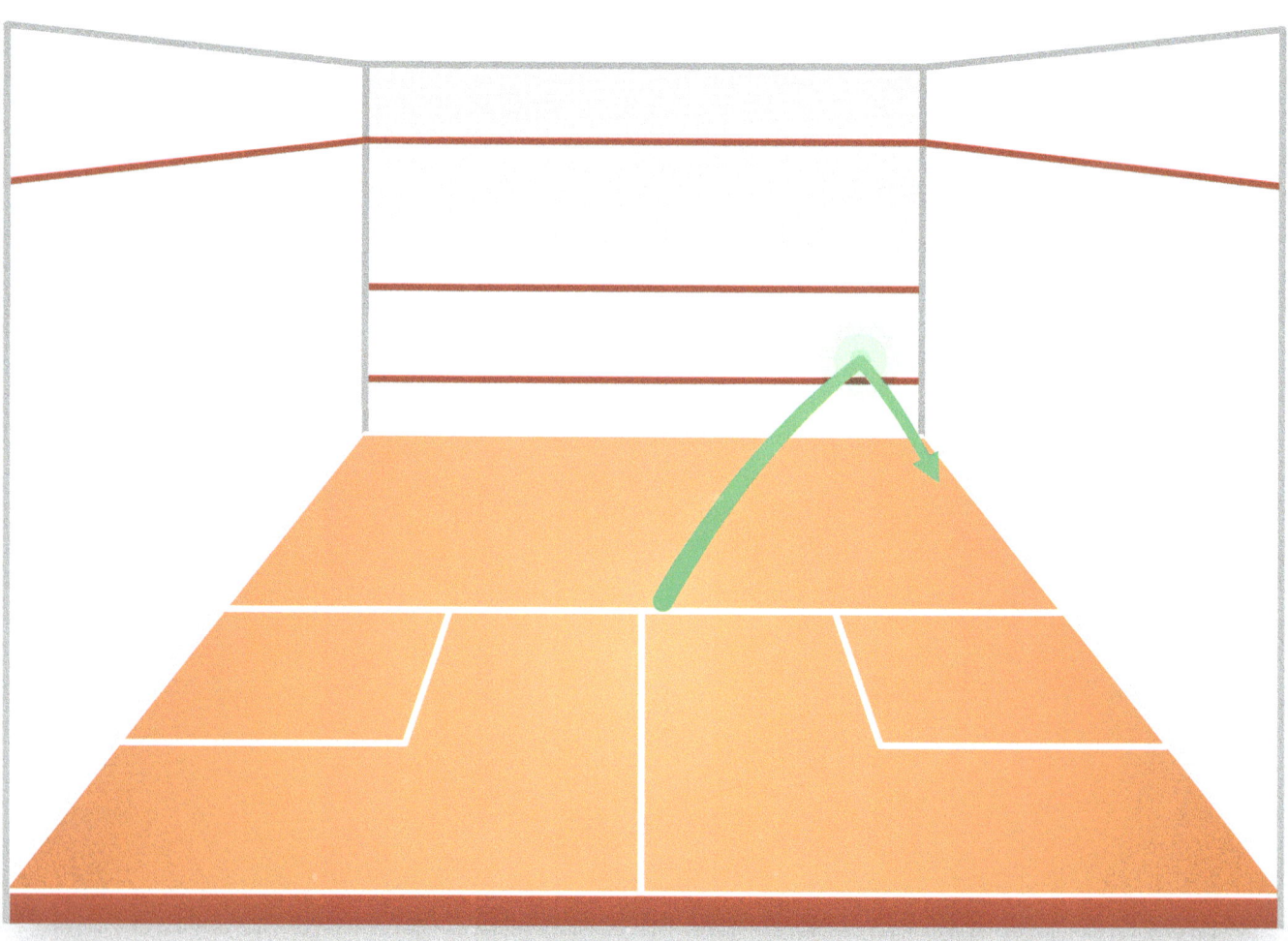

Illustration 15: Shot Type - Drop FH

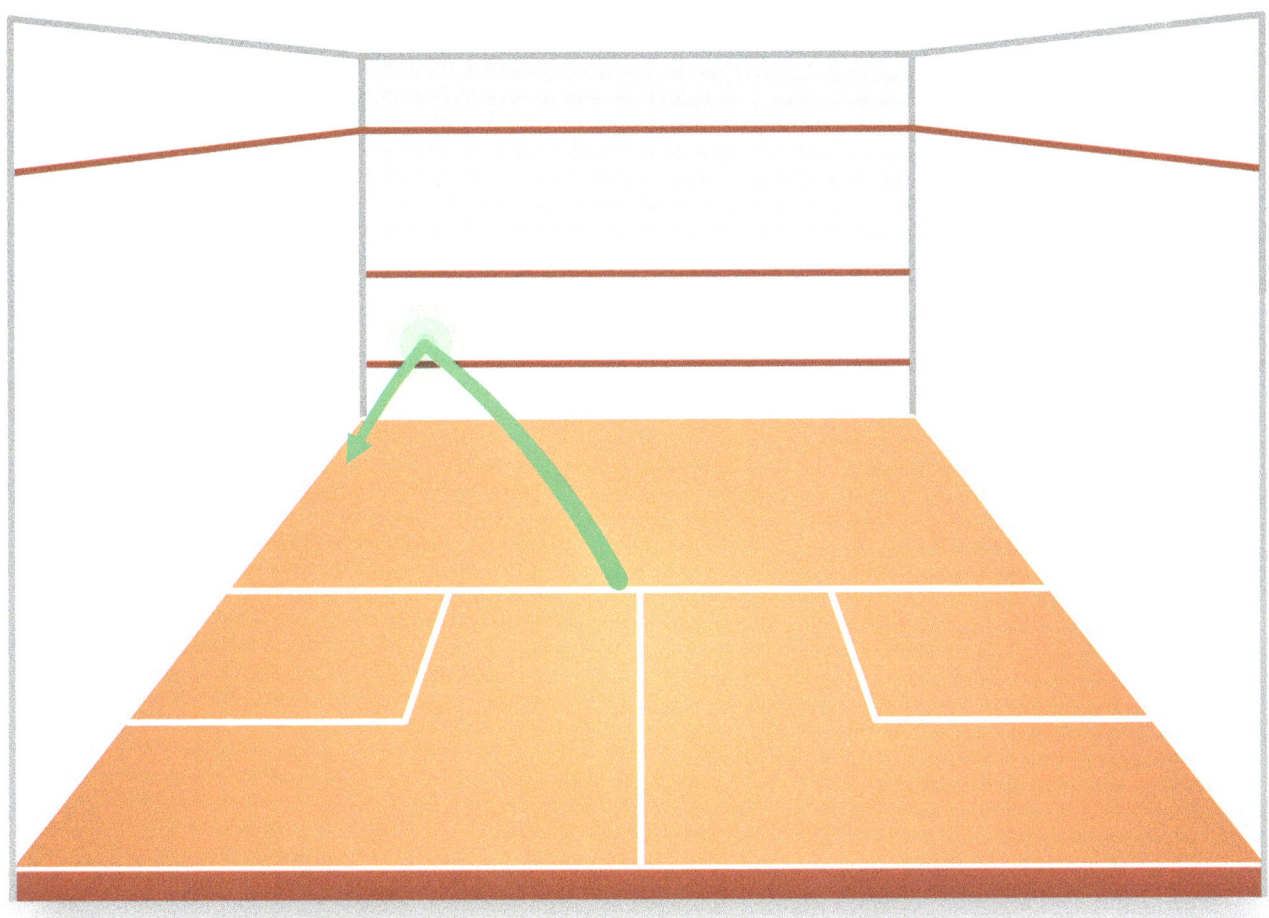

Illustration 16: Shot Type - Drop BH

Kill:

Kill shots are attacking shots, played with a lot of power on the front wall in Quarter 1 aimed just above the tin. Kill shots can be played at a medium or hard pace. The purpose of the shot is to play it nice, low and as an aggressive shot. One can play a cross court kill or a straight kill. When played as a straight kill, the aim is to hit the ball nice, low, and hard so it stays tight on the side wall, whilst the crosscourt kill is played nice, low, and hard in the middle of the front wall in Quarter 1 just above the tin, with the aim of ball bouncing more than twice before reaching the short line. In addition, it is a good tactical shot because it gets your opponent down and low when retrieving. *(Refer to Illustration 17: Shot Type - BH Straight Kill, Illustration 18: Shot Type - BH Cross Kill, Illustration 19: Shot Type - FH Straight Kill and Illustration 20: Shot Type - FH Cross Kill)*

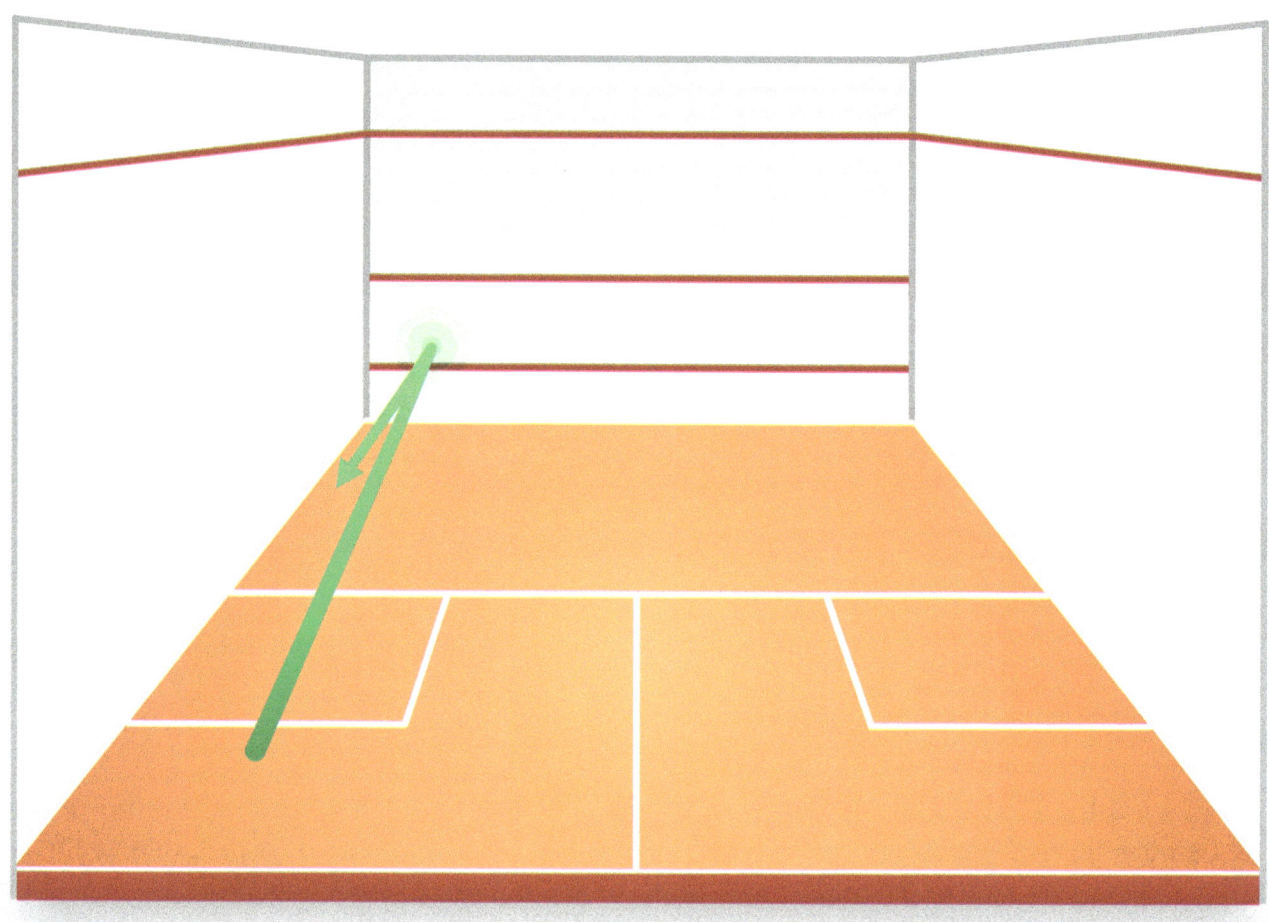

Illustration 17: Shot Type - BH Straight Kill

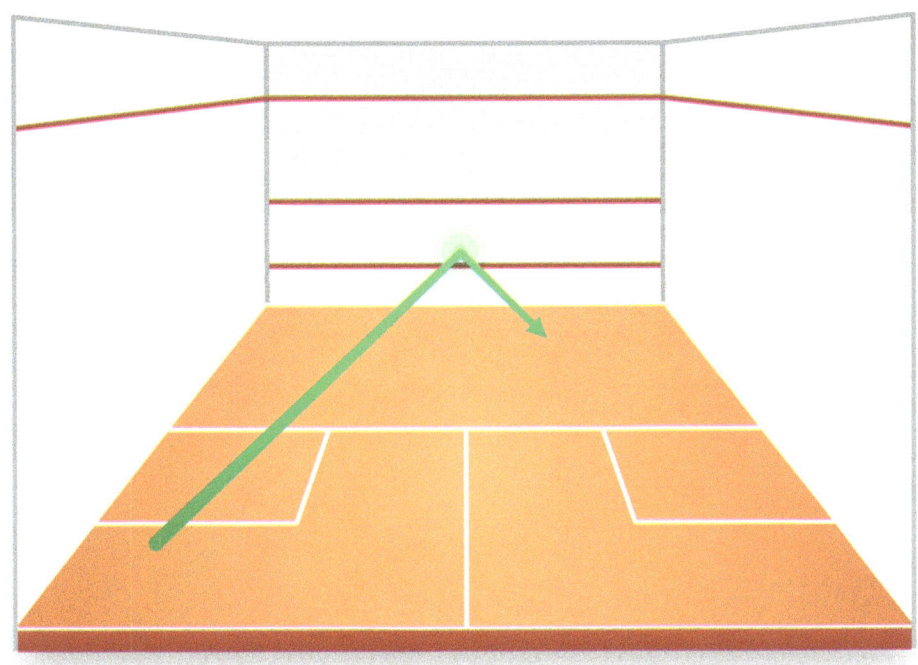

Illustration 18: Shot Type - BH Cross Kill

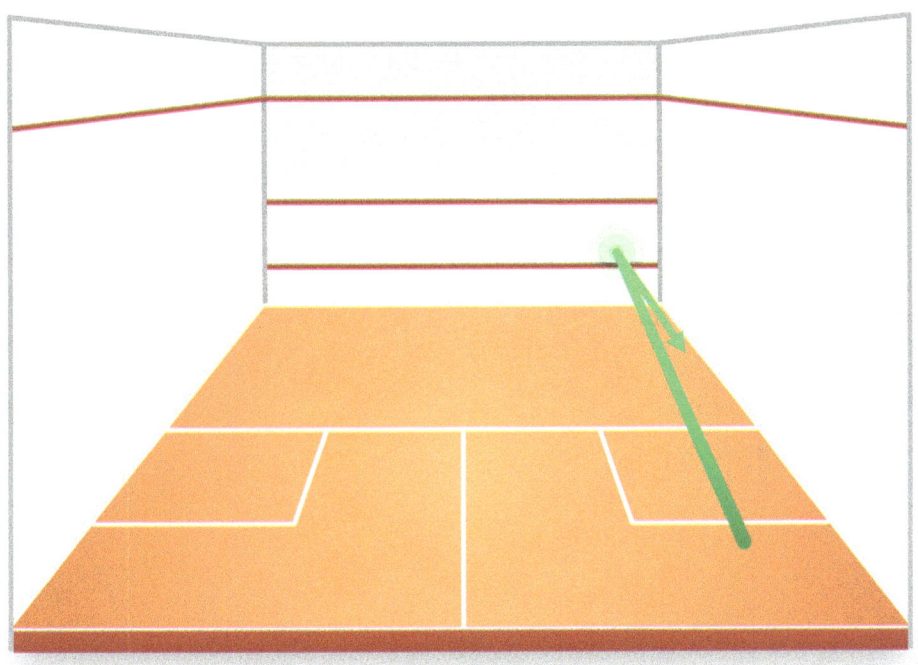

Illustration 19: Shot Type - FH Straight Kill

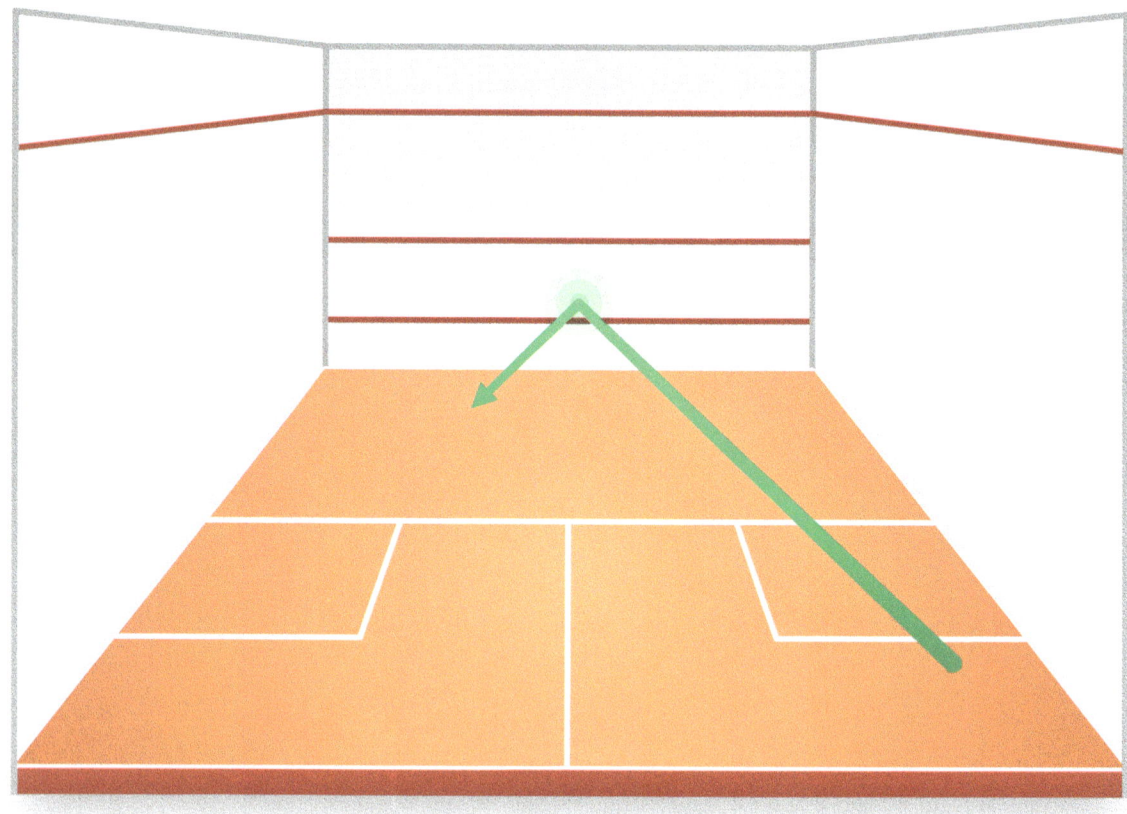

Illustration 20: Shot Type - FH Cross Kill

Lob:

There are two types of lobs that can be played: straight lobs and cross lobs. Cross lob is a soft and high shot typically played on the front wall in Quarter 4 in a way to make the ball arc. The lob aims to lift the ball as high as possible in a trajectory and getting it to land in the opposite back corner inside the pie. Straight lob, on the other hand, is played on the front wall in Quarter 4 in a way to make the ball stick along the side walls. The purpose of playing lobs is to buy one recovery time when under pressure and also to put an opponent in a vulnerable and defensive position when played as an attacking shot, because it allows one to gain the "T" position and follow up for the next shot. *(Refer to Illustration 21: Shot Type - FH Straight Lob, Illustration 22: Shot Type - FH Cross Lob, Illustration 23: Shot Type - BH Straight Lob and Illustration 24: Shot Type - BH Cross Lob)*

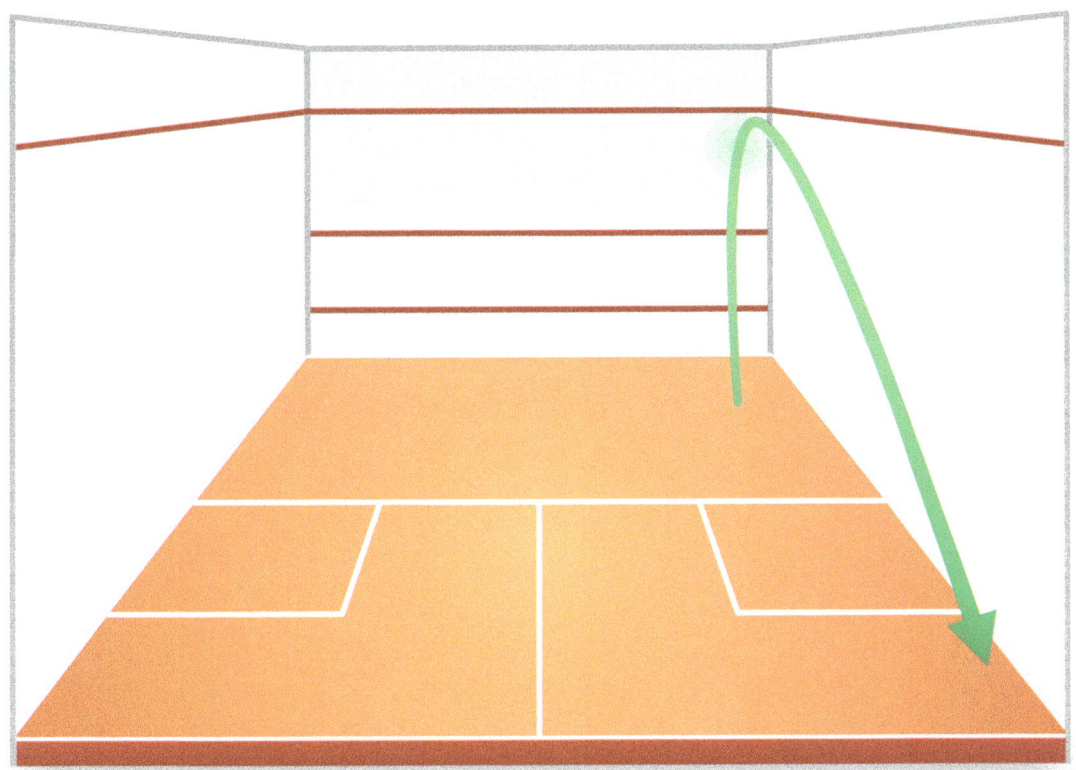

Illustration 21: Shot Type - FH Straight Lob

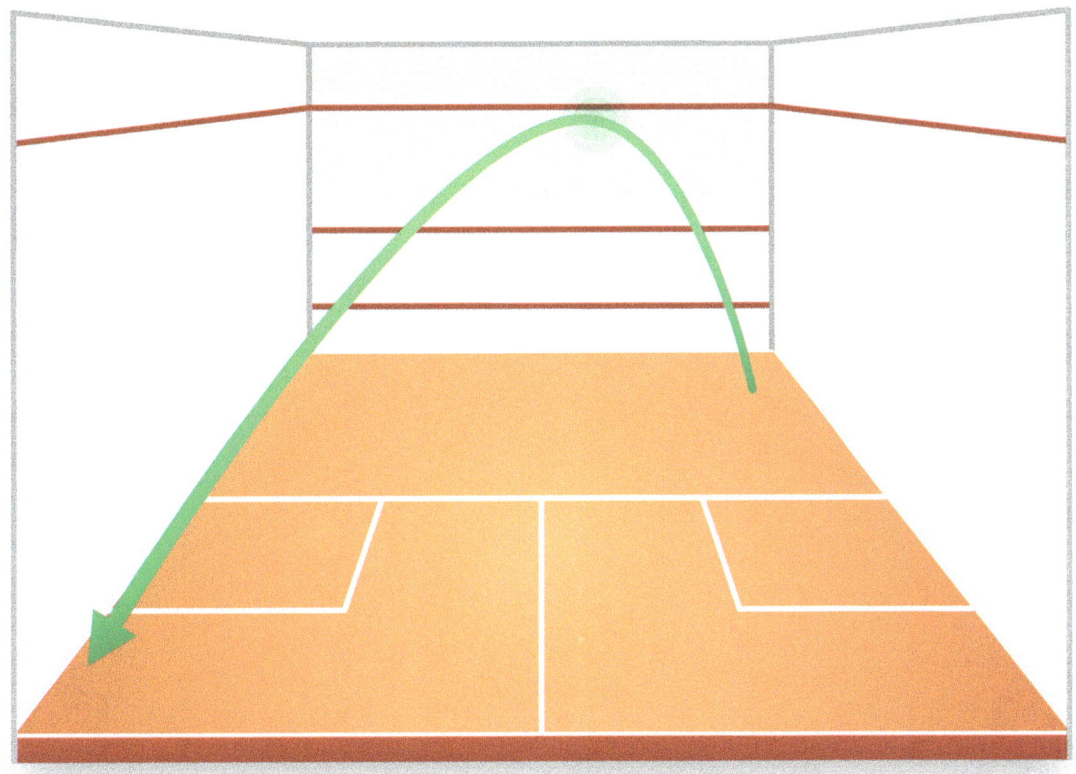

Illustration 22: Shot Type - FH Cross Lob

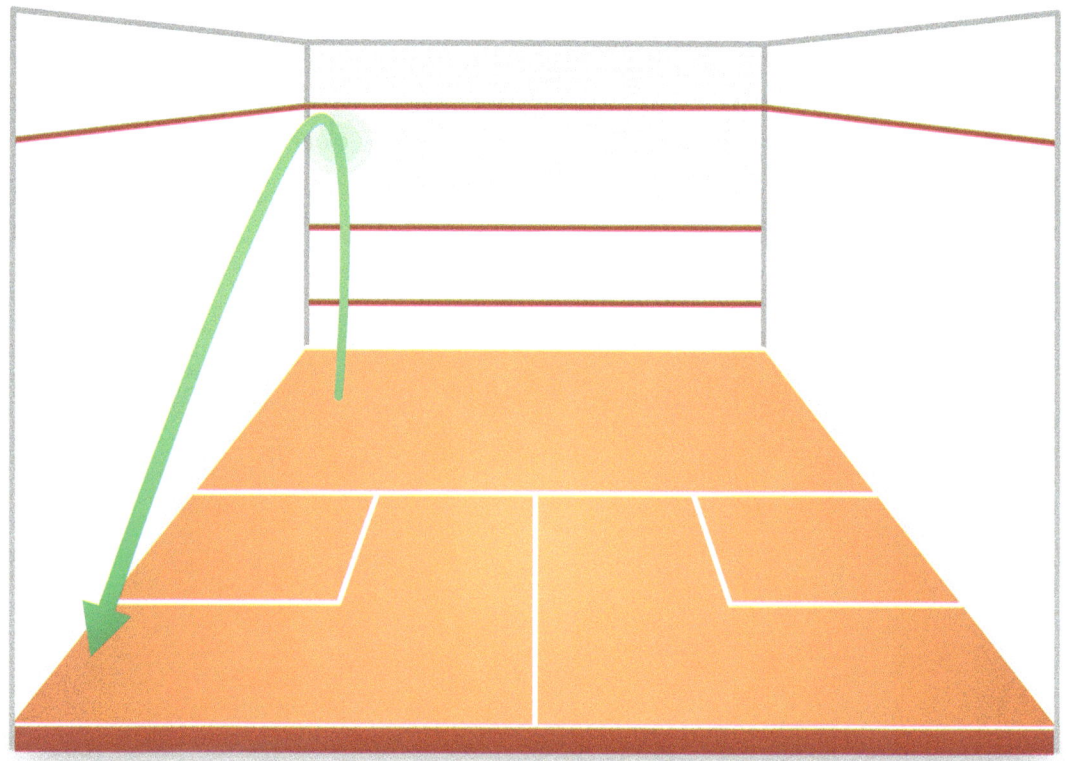

Illustration 23: Shot Type - BH Straight Lob

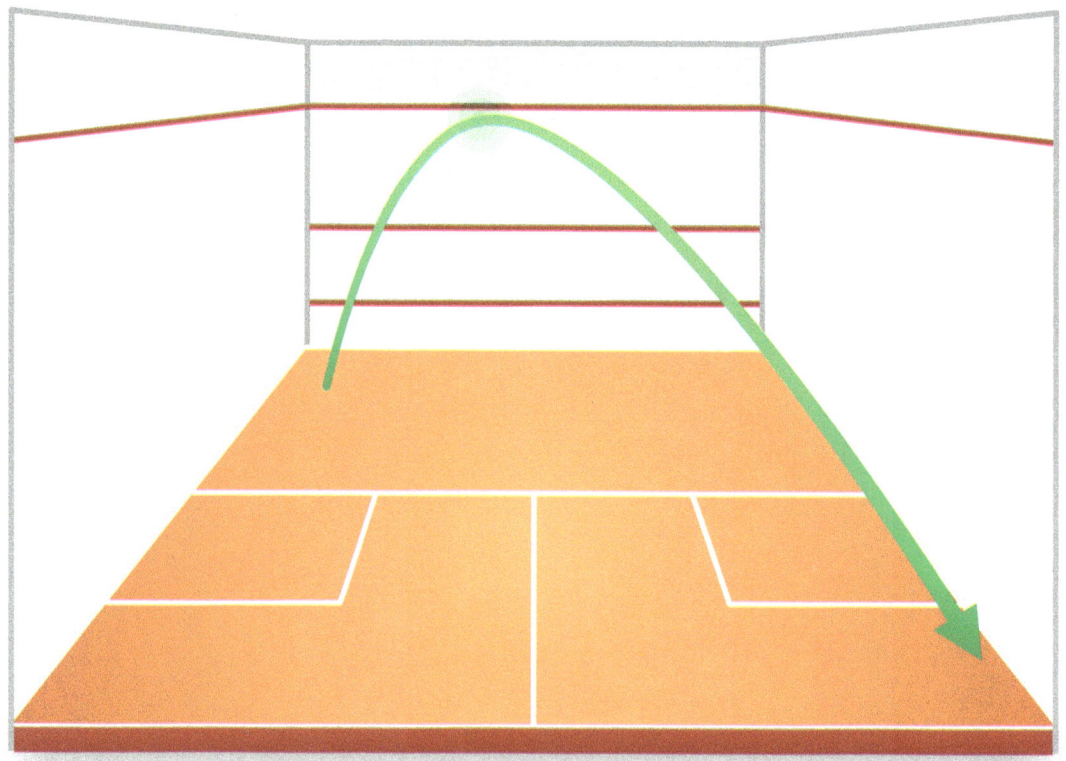

Illustration 24: Shot Type - BH Cross Lob

4.5 Types of Balls

Squash balls are made from raw butyl rubber, also known as isobutylene-isoprene rubber, combined with other natural and synthetic materials and powders to enhance the ball's performance. The rubber mixture is moulded into two hemispheres, which are then glued together to form a hollow sphere and polished to a matte finish. Squash balls come in standard sizes, with a diameter ranging from 3.95cm to 4.05cm and weighing 23g to 25g. Different types of balls are available to suit different playing styles and speeds, and the material's resilience is an important factor affecting a ball's performance. This is because resilience allows the ball to absorb and release energy. Squash balls come in six varieties, each with varying levels of bounce, indicated by coloured dots. *(Refer to Illustration 25: Types of Balls)*

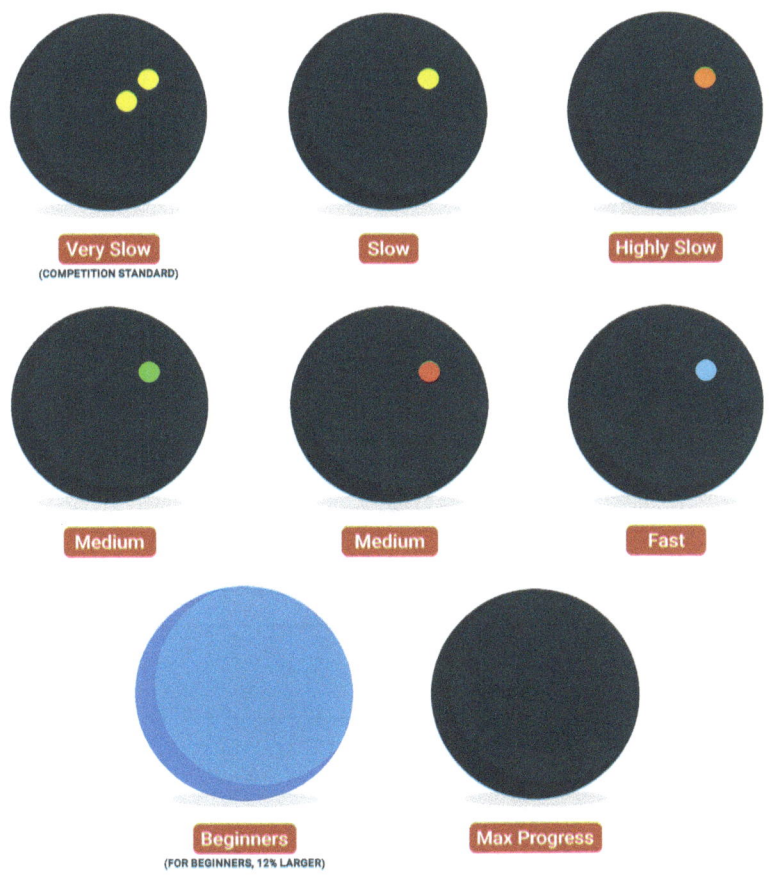

Ball Colour	Ball Speed	Ball Bounce	Level of Player
Blue	Fast	Very High	Intro/Novice
Red	Medium	High	Progress/Beginners
Green	Medium	Average	Intermediate
Single Yellow	Slow	Low	Advanced
Double Yellow	Very Slow	Very Low	Experienced/Professionals
Orange	Highly Slow	Super Low	Only of High Altitude Play

Illustration 25: Types of Balls

Full Name: _____

Date: _____

4.6 Q&A Task: Describe your understanding of the parts of the court and list all the parts that make up a squash court?

_____

_____

_____

_____

_____

_____

_____

_____

_____

_____

_____

_____

_____

_____

_____

Full Name: _____

Date: _____

4.7 **Q&A Task:** What is it meant by the below statements, and in your own words, describe the 4 Quadrants and 4 Quarters of the squash court?

> *"There are 4 Quadrants of the floor or surface area of the court, which is very important to understand as it helps one with the placement of the shots as well as movement."*

> *"The front wall of the squash court is divided into 4 Quarters (4 Qs)."*

> *"It was found that each quarter of the front wall has a purpose."*

_____

_____

_____

_____

_____

_____

_____

_____

_____

_____

Full Name: _____

Date: _____

4.8 Q&A Task: What is a common mistake that amateurs make when it comes to the Three Zones?

_____

_____

_____

_____

_____

_____

_____

_____

_____

_____

_____

_____

_____

_____

Full Name: _____

Date: _____

4.9 Q&A Task: List all the basic shot types and write what their purpose is and how can you use it?

_____

_____

_____

_____

_____

_____

_____

_____

_____

_____

_____

_____

_____

_____

Section Five

Squash Court Rules

5.1 Scoring System

There are three main types of scoring systems when it comes to squash games.

1) Hand-in-Hand-Out (HIHO) 9 points (Vintage version)
2) Point-A-Rally (PAR) 15 points (Older version)
3) Point-A-Rally (PAR) 11 points (Current version)

Hand-In-Hand-Out (HIHO) 9 Points (Vintage Version):

The first scoring system, known as Hand-In-Hand-Out (HIHO), was used prior to the introduction of Point-A-Rally (PAR) and is considered a vintage version. It is played to 9 points and in a best of 5 games format. In this system, players can only win points while serving. For example, if Player A serves and Player B receives and wins the rally, the score will not change and Player B will become the server. If Player B then wins the rally he served, he earns a point.

Point-A-Rally (PAR) 15 Points (Older Version):

The second scoring system, Point-A-Rally (PAR), was used from 1989 to 2003 and is played to 15 points in a best of 5 games format, with a tiebreak of 2 clear points at 14-14. In this format, every point counts. For example, if Player A serves and Player B receives and wins the rally, Player B earns a point and will serve.

Point-A-Rally (PAR) 11 Points (Current Version):

Starting on April 1st, 2009, the World Squash Federation (WSF) voted to change the scoring system to Point-A-Rally (PAR) played to 11 points with a tiebreak of 2 clear points at 10-10 in a best of 5 games format. This scoring format is similar to the PAR 15 points but played to 11 points. This new scoring system took effect worldwide and is used in professional squash matches by the Professional Squash Association (PSA). On occasion, matches may be played in a best of 3 games format.

5.2 Decisions for Refereeing

In a squash game, players aim to control their movements, but it's common for them to obstruct each other's path to the ball accidentally. To resolve these incidents, there are set rules in place.

These rules consist of the "Let," "No Let," and "Stroke" decisions.

Let

A "Let" decision means the rally will be played again, as the interference was accidental, and both players made their best effort to continue the rally.

No Let

A "No Let" decision means the point is awarded to the player who struck the ball and provided clear access, as the interference was minimal. The referee makes this decision after considering the situation.

Stroke

A "Stroke" decision means the point is awarded to the player who appealed and stopped playing the ball due to the other player's obstruction. The player who caused the obstruction by playing a loose shot is at fault.

Both players have a responsibility to provide clear access to the ball and allow their opponent to play a shot without any obstruction. If a player believes that interference has occurred, they can request a "Let" from the referee. If there's no referee, the players must come to a mutual agreement on the ruling based on the circumstances.

5.3 How to Start the Play

Toss (Spinning of Racket):

To start the match, both players will do a spin of the racket which is similar to a coin toss. When spinning a racket, a player is asked to choose either up or down and/or left or right depending on the logo. The purpose of spinning the racket is to pick a winner who will serve first.

Starting a Rally:

After the toss, a winner is picked. The first shot that a player will hit is the serve. To serve, a player must always keep one foot inside the service box when going through the serving motion. A player can pick which side he would like to serve either at the start of the match or after winning each rally. A player can choose to serve from the left side service box or (Quadrant 3) or right-side service box (Quadrant 4). In addition, when serving, the ball must hit the front wall either in Quarter 3 or 4 or between the service line and outline with the aim of getting the ball landed on the opposite part of the court behind the front or short line. Once the shot is finished, the player serving must return to the "T" and control the "T" position. *(Refer to Illustration 26: Serve from Right Service Box and Illustration 27: Serve from Left Service Box)*

On the other hand, the player retrieving the serve must stand just behind the service box opposite the quadrant of the player serving. The player can choose to either volley the serve after it hits the front wall or let it bounce once before hitting it. It is important for a retriever to first look to volley the serve. If it is difficult to volley, then the player can look to hit it off the bounce.

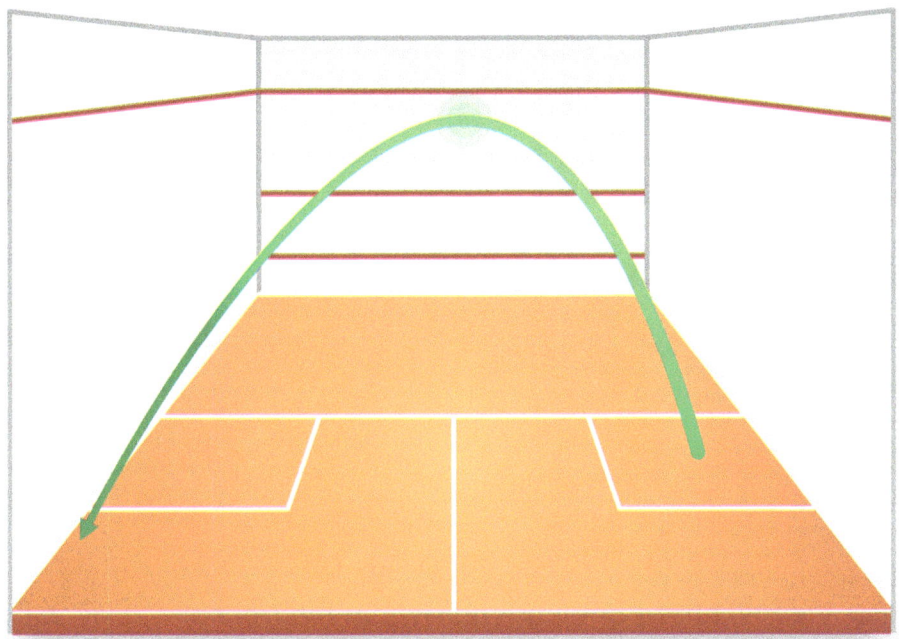

Illustration 26: Serve from Right Service Box

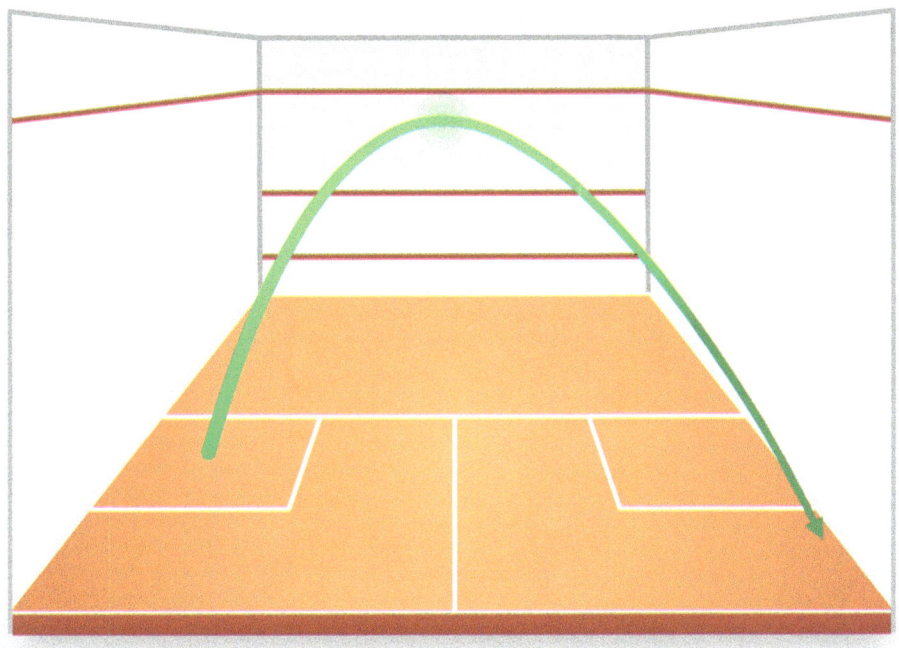

Illustration 27: Serve from Left Service Box

Constructing a Rally:

The basic axiom of a squash rally is to take turns hitting the ball against the front wall until a player is unable to retrieve the shot. This can occur if the ball is too close to the side wall, bounces twice, goes out of bounds, hits the tin or floor, or if the player strikes the ball more than once. The ball must travel to the front wall after each shot.

A player is allowed to let the ball bounce once on the floor and multiple times on the side or back walls before returning the shot. It's crucial for a player to get back to the "T" after each shot and maintain control of the position by volleying and cutting their opponent's shots on the front or short line.

By applying the principles in preceding section *(Two 4s)*, a player can strategically use the 4 Quarters on the front wall and 4 Quadrants to win rallies.

Winning a Rally and Gaining a Point:

To win a rally and gain points, some sets of rules must be followed. A player can gain a point when an opponent either:

1) Serves under or on the service line or on the outlines of the front wall, side walls or back wall
2) Hits the ball on the second bounce
3) Hits the ball above or on the outlines of the front wall, side walls or back wall
4) Hits the ball into the tin or floor or surface area of the court
5) Makes a connection with the ball more than once when striking
6) Hits the ball to a player's body or their clothing
7) Referee or players agree to a No let or Stroke ruling in situations.

Full Name: _____

Date: _____

5.4 **Q&A Task:** In your own words, define the three main types of the scoring system using the below statement as a guide:

"There are three main types of the scoring system when it comes to squash games.

1) Hand-in-Hand-Out (HIHO) 9 points (Vintage version)
2) Point-A-Rally (PAR) 15 points (Older version)
3) Point-A-Rally (PAR) 11 points (Current version)"

_____

_____

_____

_____

_____

_____

_____

_____

_____

_____

_____

_____

Full Name: _____

Date: _____

5.5   **Q&A Task:** Write an essay describing this statement and give examples of Let, No Let and Stroke. You can make up a scenario or use a scenario that you have personally experienced:

"The referee then assesses the situation and will make a decision of Let, No Let or Stroke. In instances, where there are no referees present, then both the players must come to an agreement of what ruling they should accept subject to the circumstance."

_____

_____

_____

_____

_____

_____

_____

_____

_____

_____

_____

_____

Full Name: _____

Date: _____

5.6 **Q&A Task:** In your own words, define why the statement below is true?

*"It is very wise for a player to apply the principles in the preceding section **(Two 4s)** because a player can use the 4 Quarters on the front wall and the 4 Quadrants to strategically construct and win rallies."*

_____

_____

_____

_____

_____

_____

_____

_____

_____

_____

_____

_____

Section Six

Fundamentals of Technique

6.1 The Grip

The squash racket grip is one of the most basic, important, and neglected parts of a squash technique, whether it's on the forehand (FH) or backhand (BH). Any level of player must grasp an understanding of how to hold the squash racket correctly. It is these basic steps that can help one further improve their technique.

Handshake grip or V Shape grip:

Handshake grip, also known as a V Shape grip, is the correct way to hold a squash racket grip. The name itself is quite simple to understand, but it is the most misunderstood. The steps to follow when correctly holding the squash racket grip are as follows. Follow each step thoroughly, as it is one of the first and most fundamental steps when it comes to the squash technique

1) Hold your racket out in front of you straight with the handle facing you and shake one hand with your racket grip
2) Relax your grip between thumb and index finger
3) Use your remaining three fingers to give support to your grip
4) Avoid squeezing the handle and connecting thumb and fingers together
5) This should form a V shape alignment with inside grip line of racket shaft
6) Semi-lock your wrist next by lifting the racket up slightly
7) Tilt your racket face back a little to open the racket face. ***(Refer to Illustration 28: FH Grip and Illustration 29: BH Grip)***

The racket grip stays the same on the forehand and backhand side. The racket grip needs to be adaptable to allow one to have it open or neutral on the forehand or backhand side. Holding the racket grip correctly is an essential part when it comes to striking the ball and how the racket is facing, i.e., is it open faced, closed faced or neutral. Having the racket face open allows one to have control of the ball and offers other options. The open racket face can really help one to play quality balls, whether at the front or back of the court. It also allows one to get the strings on the ball. It gives one the ability to cut the ball, hit inside or outside of the ball, and it helps one get the ball to fade or die in the corners. Lastly, it gives one various options such as hitting short or long, high or low, etc.

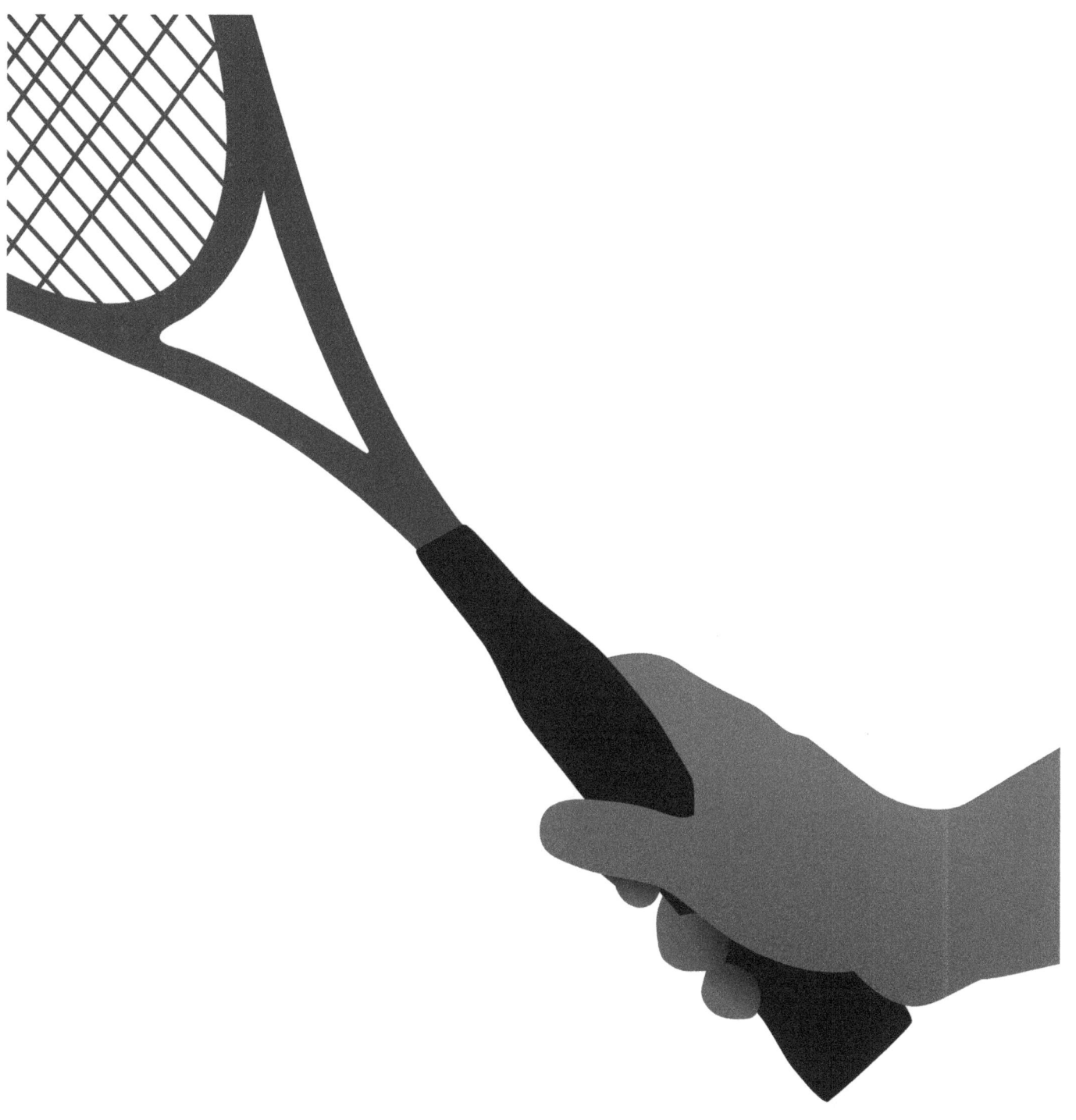

Forehand Grip

Illustration 28: FH Grip

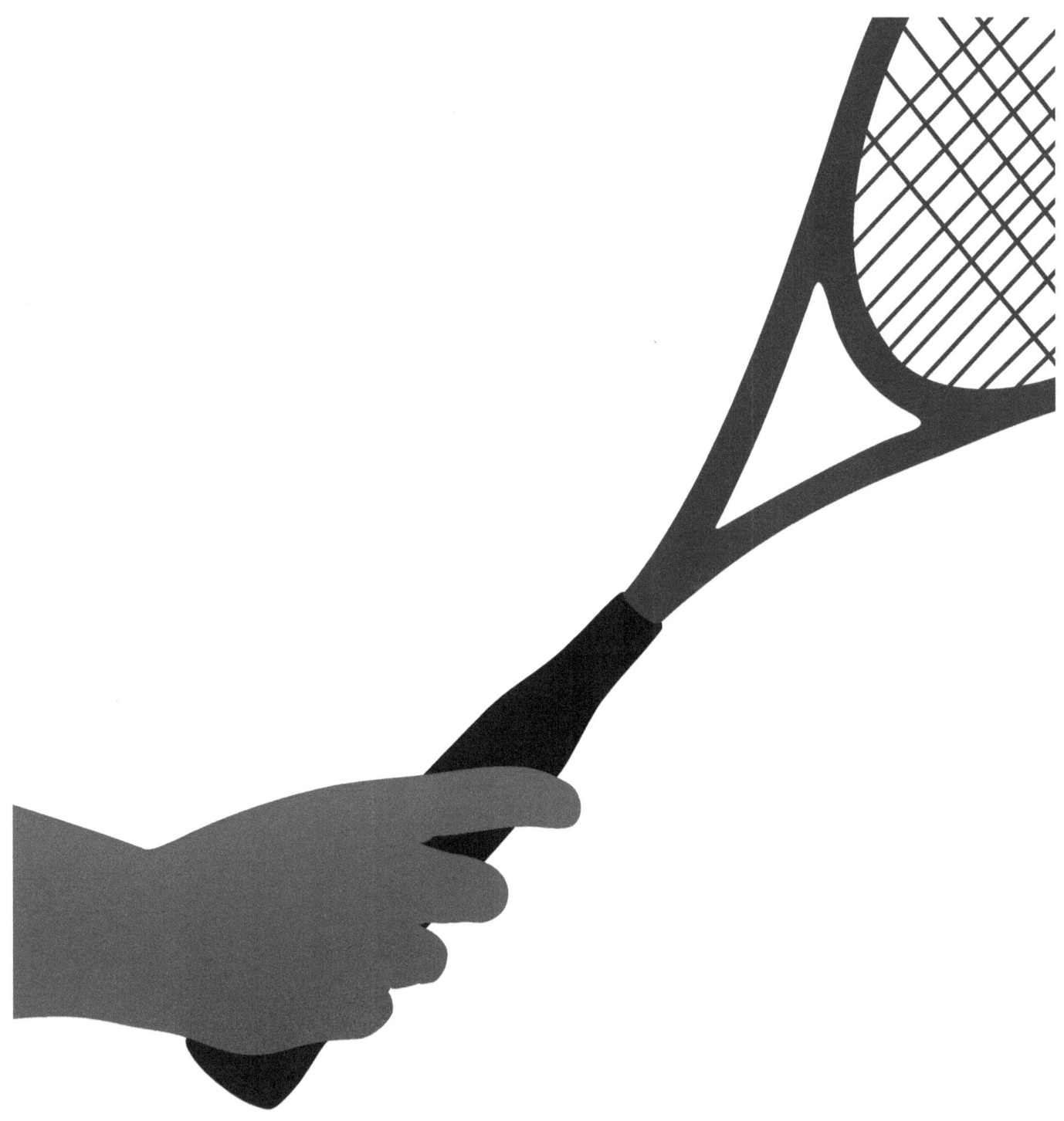

Backhand Grip

Illustration 29: BH Grip

6.2 Stages of the Technique

When it comes to the technique, whether it is forehand (FH) or backhand (BH), the aim should always be for the technique to look the same because it gives one an ability to create options when playing the shots. There are three stages of technique: preparation of the racket from the "T", movement and lunging to the ball and striking of the ball.

Preparation of the racket from the "T" is one of the most crucial parts of striking a clean ball. Without solid preparation, one cannot move and strike a clean ball because one won't have the time due to the racket not being prepared and in the right position. Therefore, it is vital to improve the racket's preparation so the other two stages of the technique can flow swiftly. To apply the three stages of the technique, one must follow the below steps in sequence:

1) Be on the "T" nice and neutral which means one is on their toes on the "T" with body facing the front wall, knees slightly bent and forward with racket up in front of him/her pointing to the front wall
2) Always track or watch the ball by keeping your eye on the ball
3) Take the racket back with the wrist semi-locked, do quick split step, and move from the "T" into the relevant corner
4) When approaching the ball, position yourself with right distance from the ball (typically about a racket length space)
5) Select the striking foot and make sure the body is behind the ball and in front of you
6) Step into the shot also known as transferring weight into the shot using dominant foot, turn your body so your upper body is facing the side wall which helps with squaring yourself resulting in giving you nice rotation
7) When striking the ball, make sure that you get down on the ball (lunging), let the racket head go first through the ball and upper body staying squared or facing the wall when striking. The shoulder must not open up too early
8) Follow through the ball. Follow through is crucial because it's a way of guiding the ball where you want it
9) After striking the ball, move smoothly off the shot with the aim of giving your opponent clear access to the ball. *(Refer to Illustrations 30 to 36: Steps 1 to 7 – Stages of Techniques FH) and (Refer to Illustrations 37 to 42: Steps 1 to 6 – Stages of Techniques BH)*

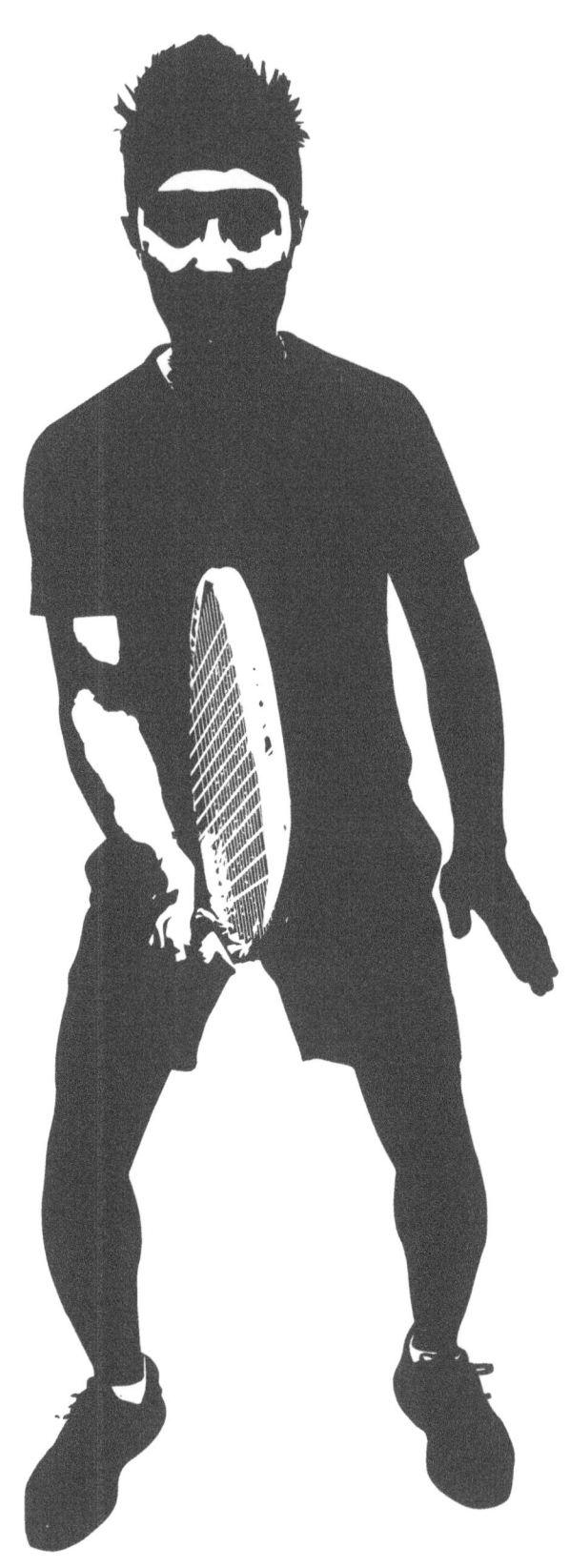

Illustration 30: Step 1 - Stages of Technique FH

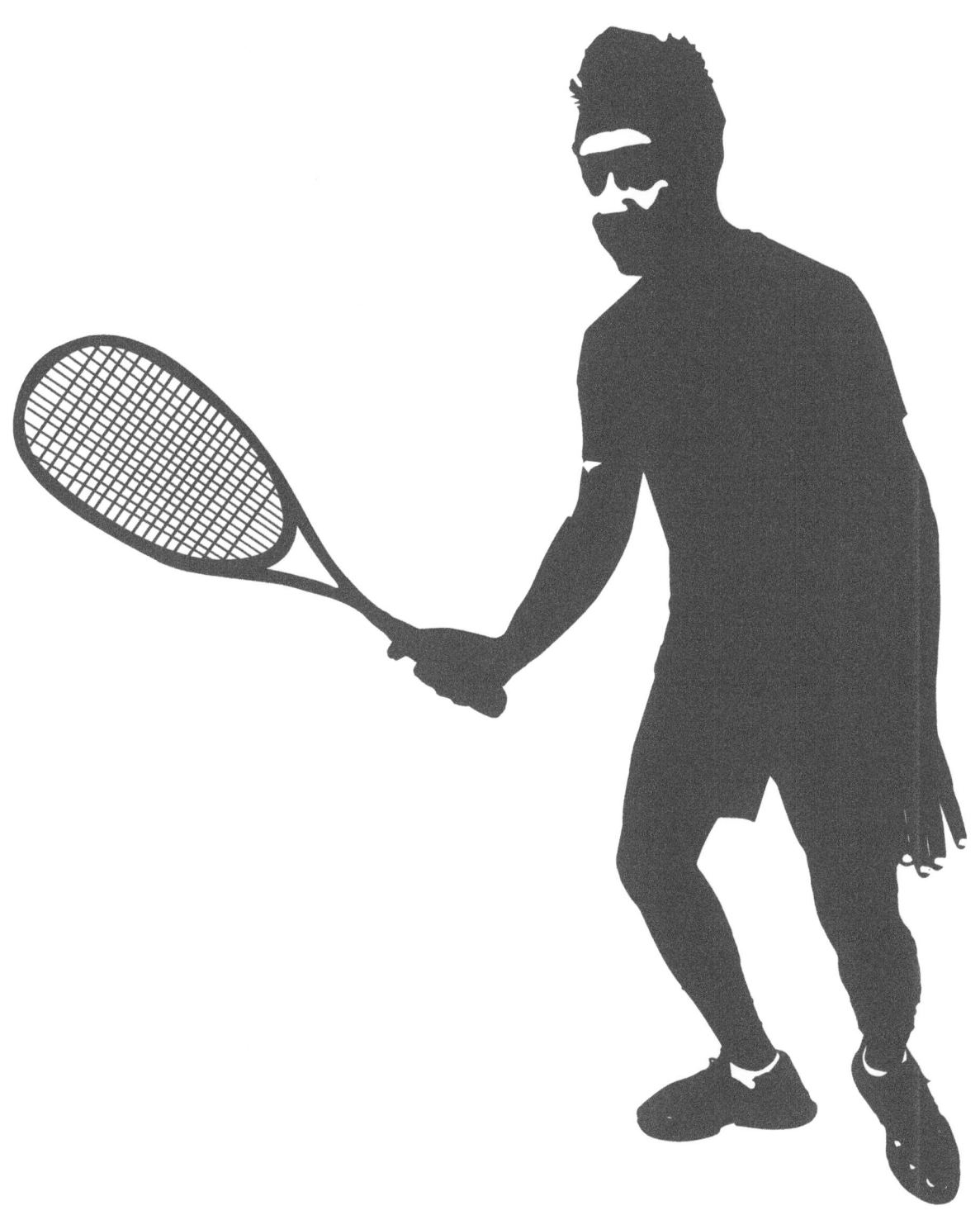

Illustration 31: Step 2 - Stages of Technique FH

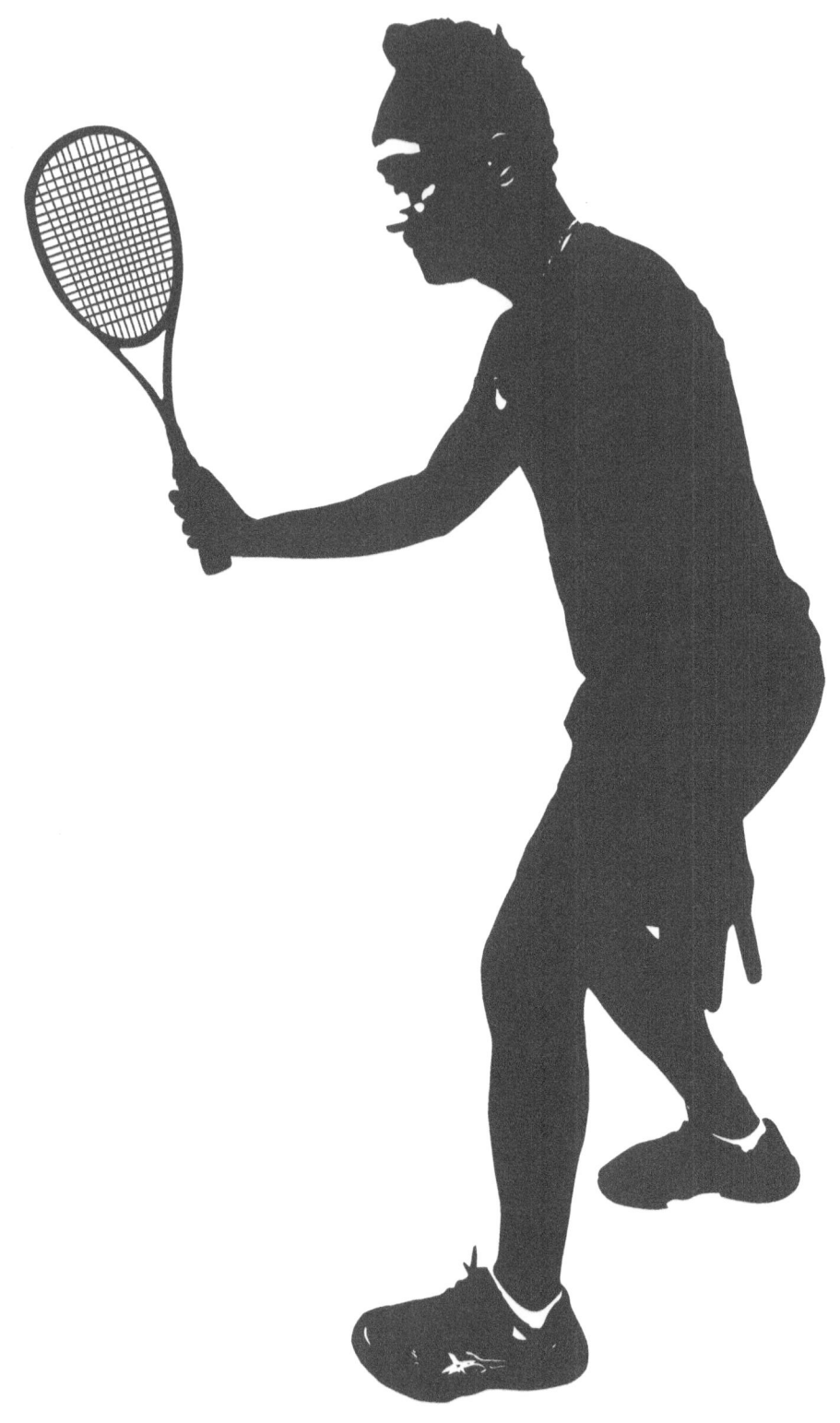

Illustration 32: Step 3 - Stages of Technique FH

Illustration 33: Step 4 - Stages of Technique FH

FUNDAMENTAL GUIDE TO BECOMING THE BEST SQUASH PLAYER

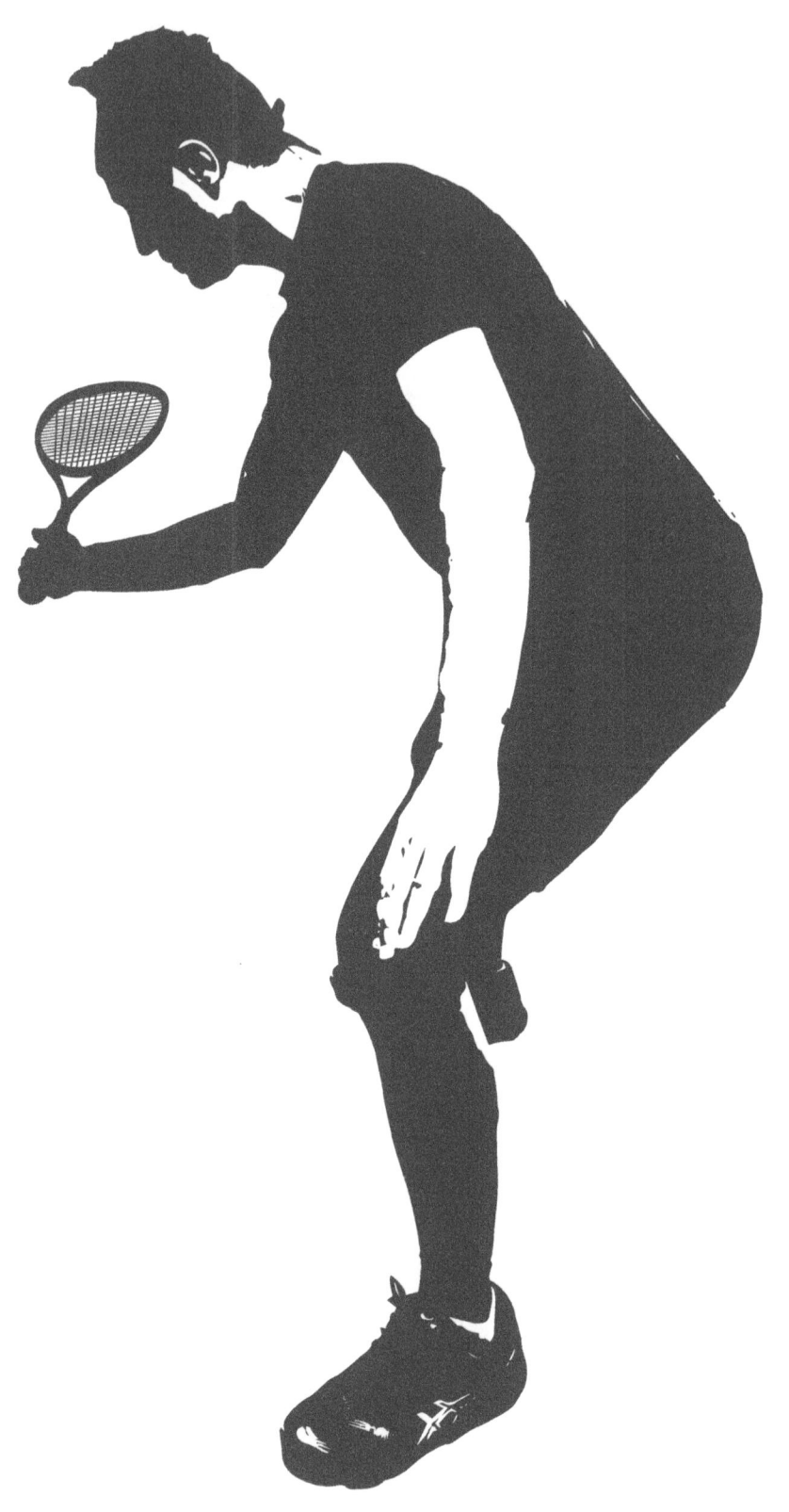

Illustration 34: Step 5 - Stages of Technique FH

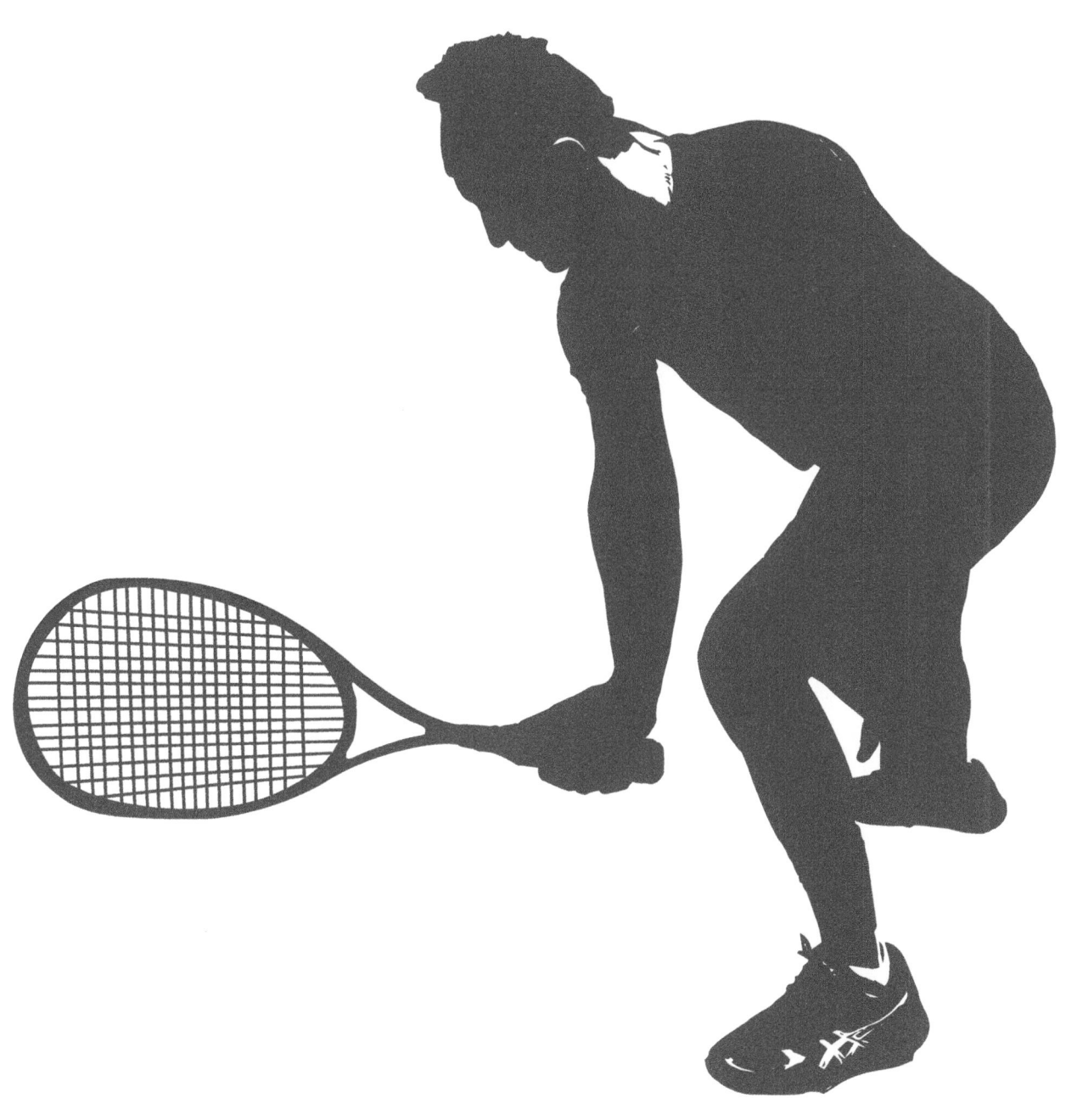

Illustration 35: Step 6 - Stages of Technique FH

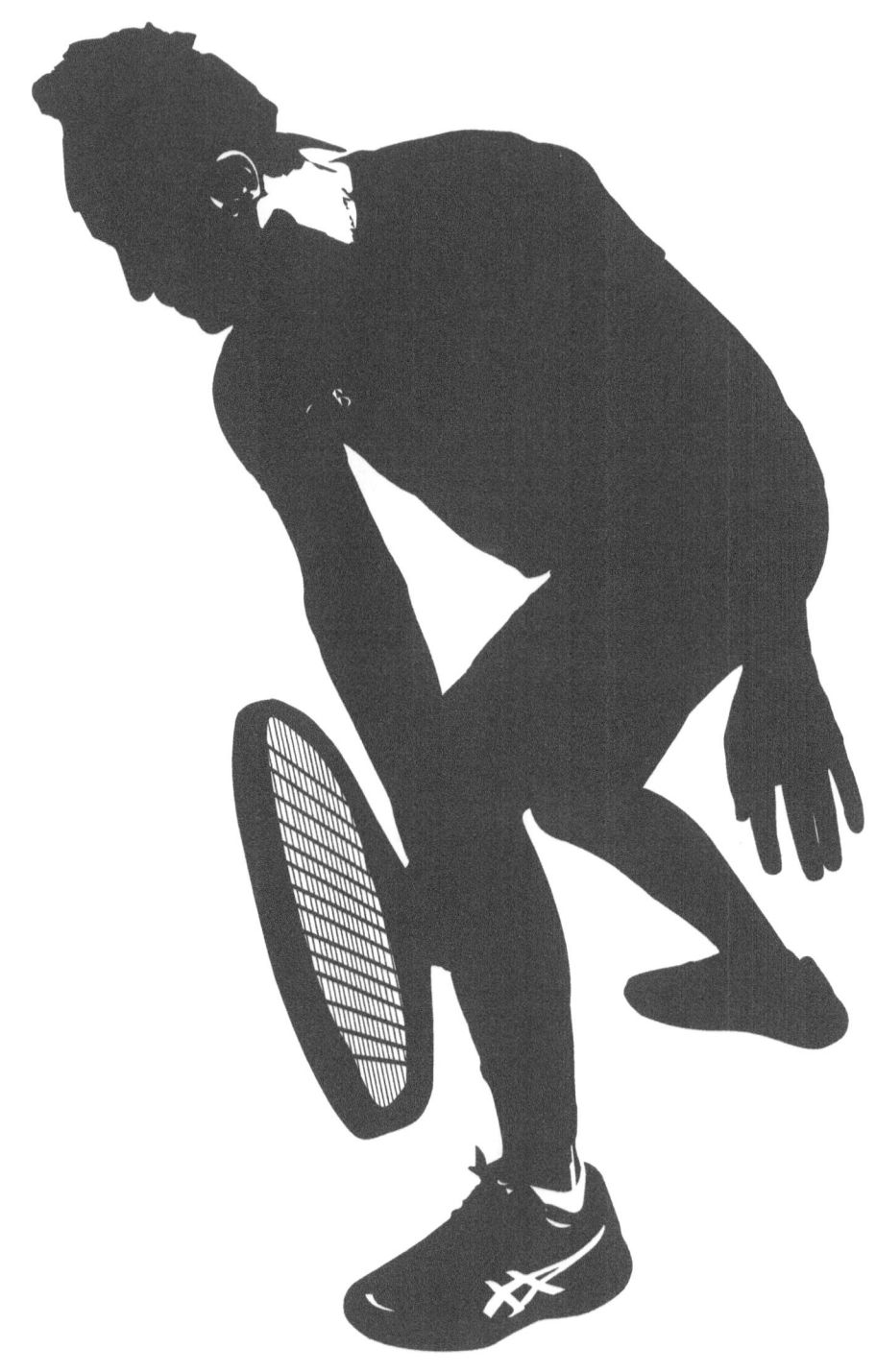

Illustration 36: Step 7 - Stages of Technique FH

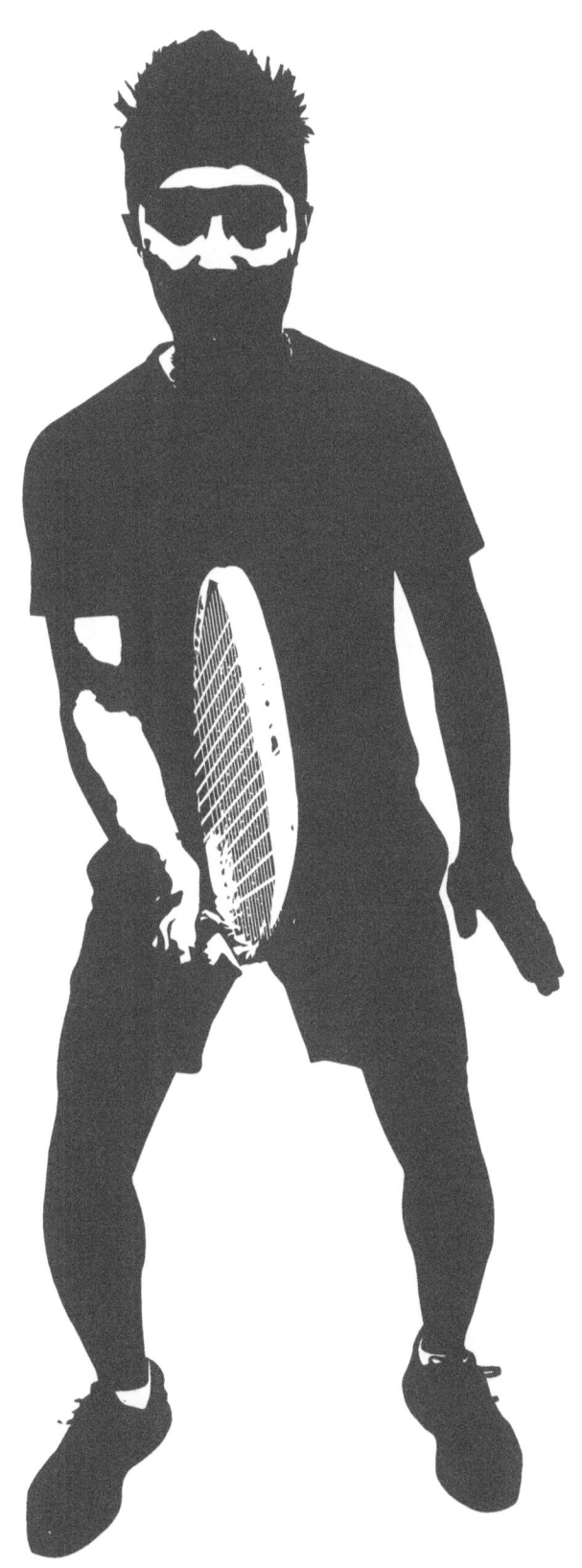

Illustration 37: Step 1 - Stages of Technique BH

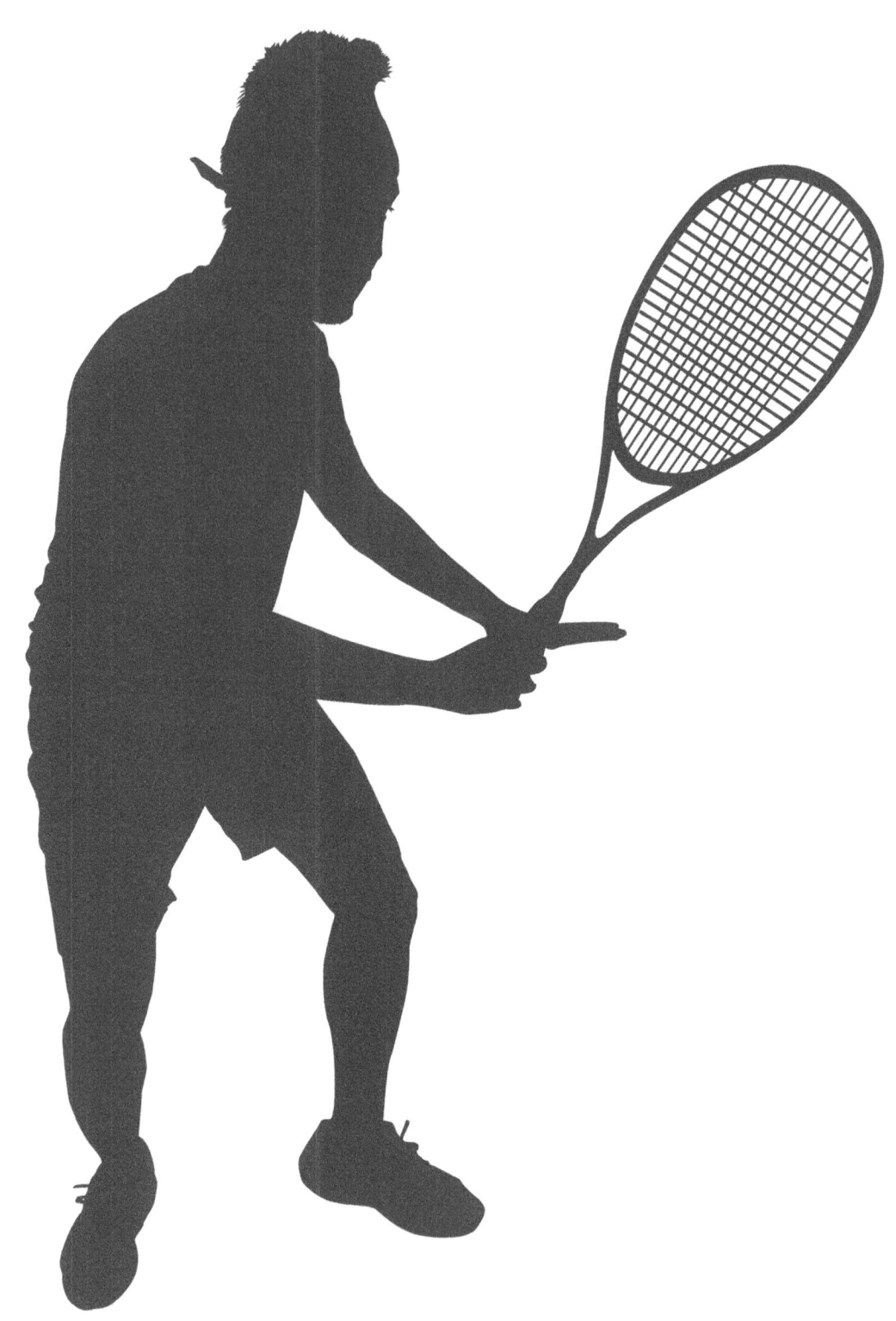

Illustration 38: Step 2 - Stages of Technique BH

FUNDAMENTAL GUIDE TO BECOMING THE BEST SQUASH PLAYER

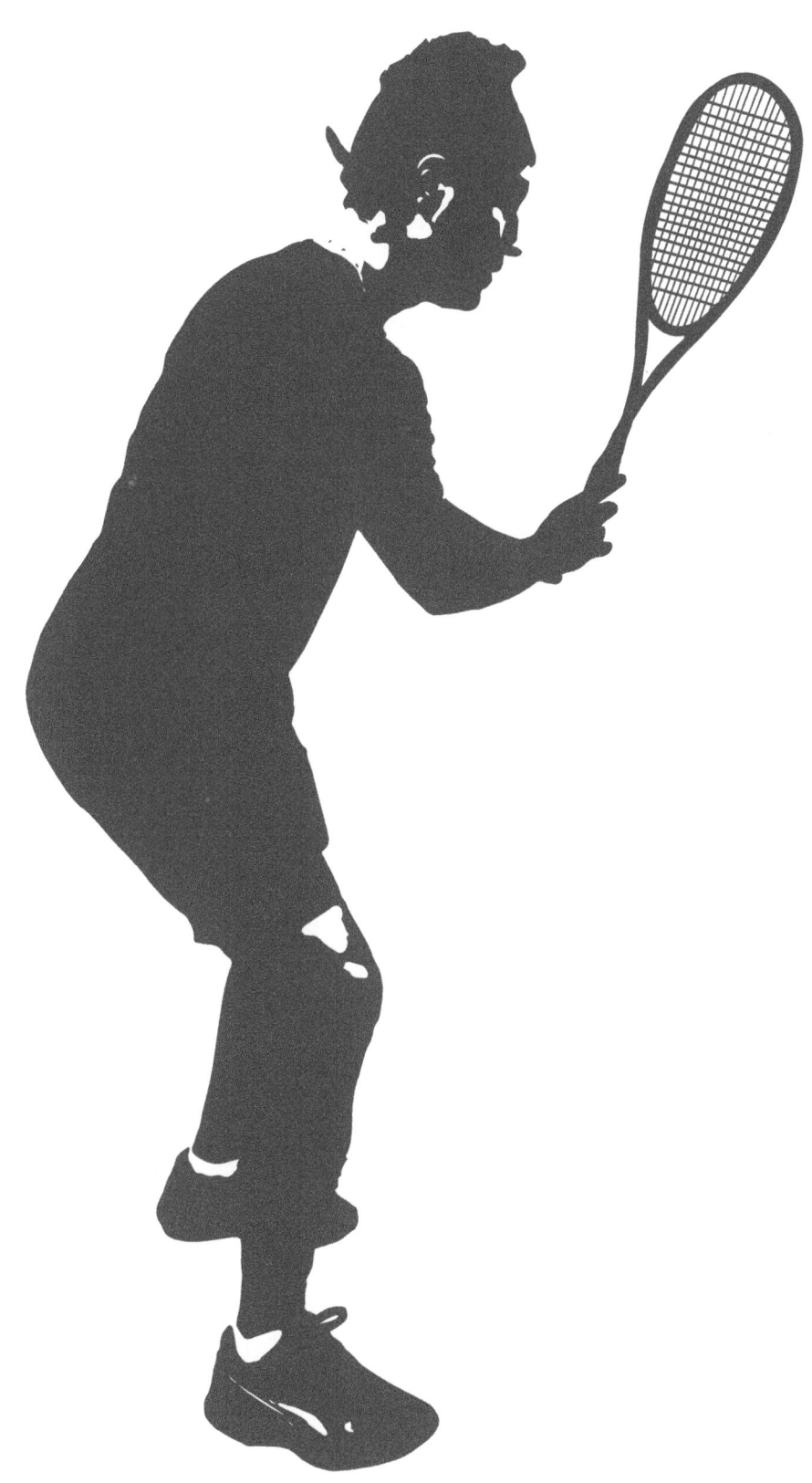

Illustration 39: Step 3 - Stages of Technique BH

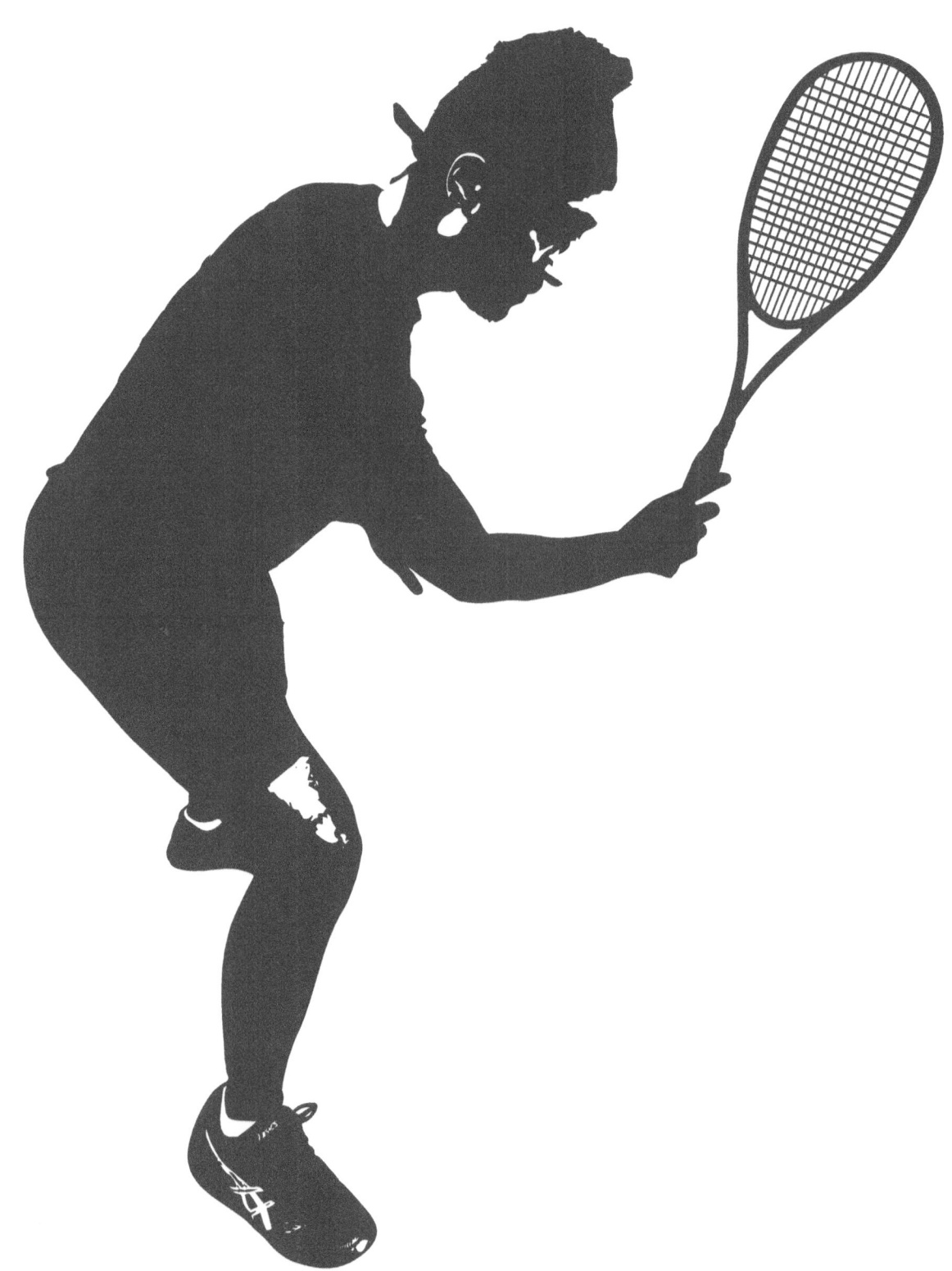

Illustration 40: Step 4 - Stages of Technique BH

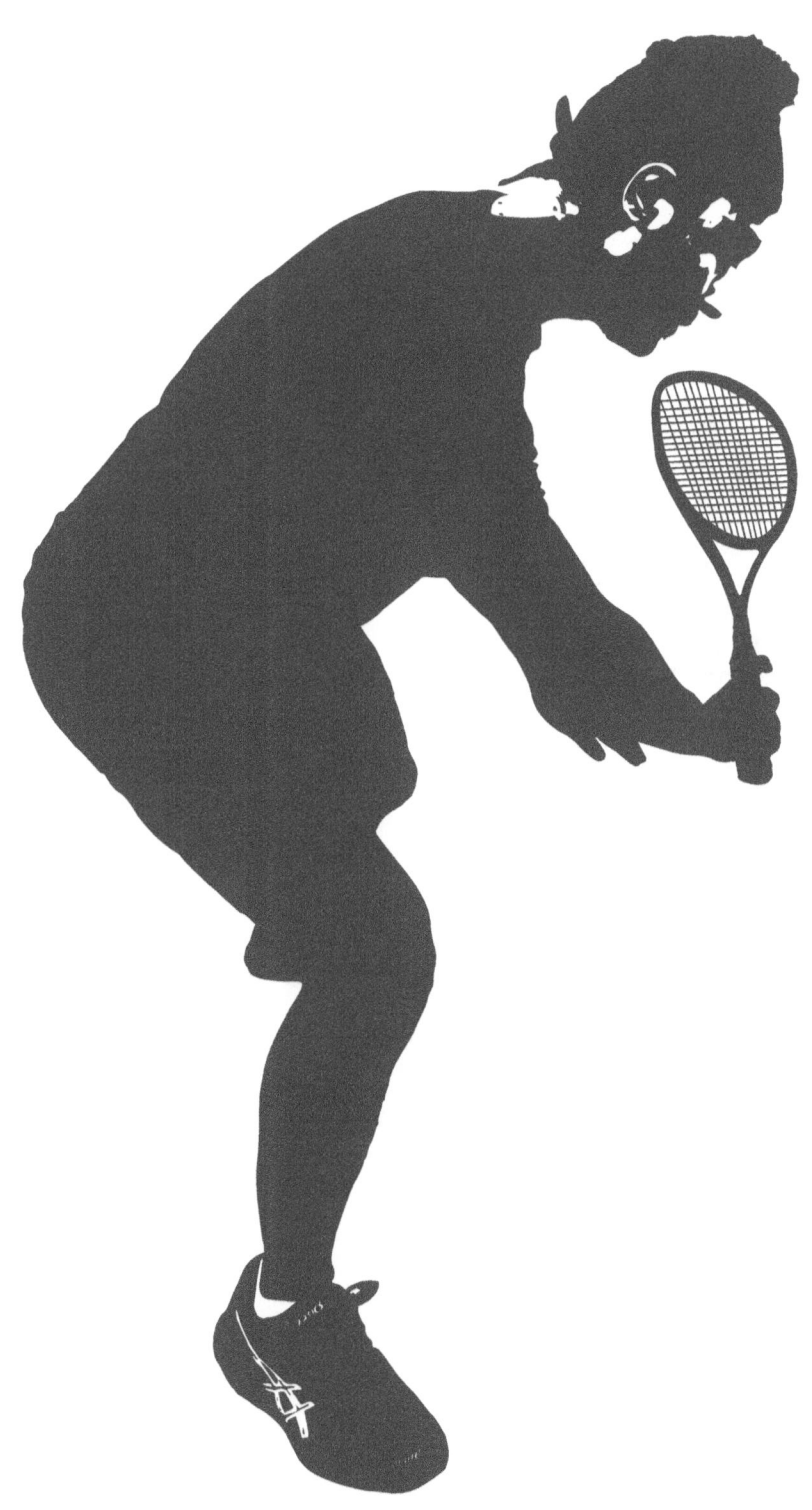

Illustration 41: Step 5 - Stages of Technique BH

FUNDAMENTAL GUIDE TO BECOMING THE BEST SQUASH PLAYER

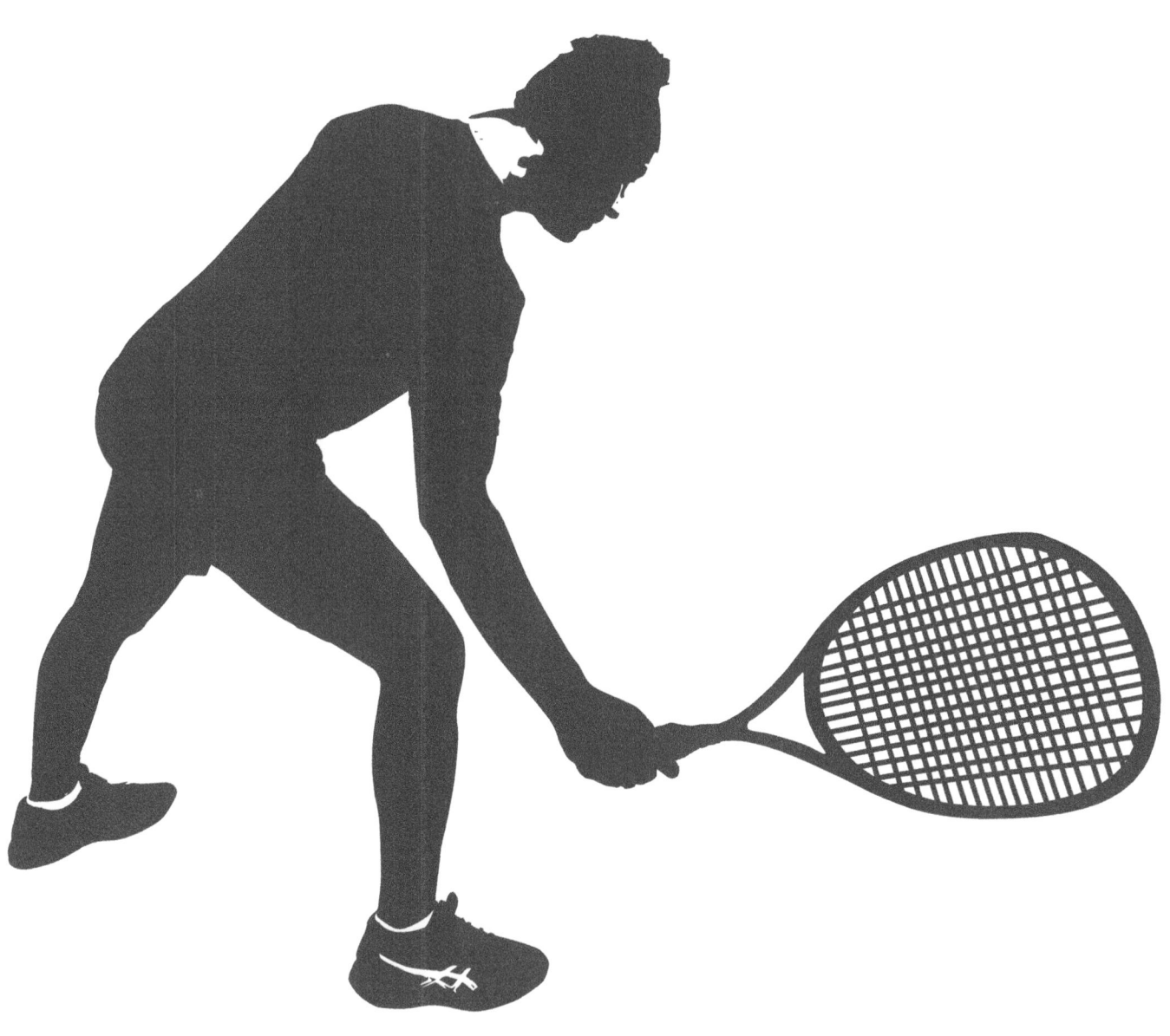

Illustration 42: Step 6 - Stages of Technique BH

Forehand (FH) and Backhand (BH) technique:

It is important to have a proper grip on the racket for both the forehand (FH) and backhand (BH) technique. The ideal position is to have the racket up and back, with a comfortable amount of space between the elbow and rib cage. The racket should not be too far away or too close to the body but somewhere in between for balance. Imagine standing on the "T" and facing the front wall. Now take the racket up and back either FH or BH so the racket head is pointing up and away at the corner without locking the wrist or relaxing it too much. It must be balanced because balance is the key. The general rule of thumb when it comes to FH or BH technique is that it should feel right and comfortable, meaning the racket up and back positioned in the middle, semi-locked wrist, racket head a little open, so the strings are facing the front wall when on the "T". In conclusion, it's essential to find a comfortable preparation position for the racket, with a slightly open racket, semi-locked wrist, and elbow slightly in, to allow for maximum swing freedom.

More on Forehand (FH) and Backhand (BH) technique:

The forehand technique in squash can be visualised by the act of skipping a stone into a river. Similar to skipping a stone, the forehand swing involves lifting the racket above the shoulder, transferring weight and stepping in, using the elbow to drive the shot, and releasing the racket to hit the ball. The forehand technique can be broken down into four key steps for better understanding and execution:

1) Racket up and back
2) Step into the shot and maintain balance
3) Get the elbow leading the swing
4) Follow through the ball, guiding it on the line where you want the ball to go whilst utilising balance in the lunge to control the shot.

On the other hand, when it comes to backhand technique, follow the five steps below:

1) Get your racket up and hold it slightly back
2) Maintain a semi-locked wrist position and make sure to adjust your shoulder in a starting position, so it sits under your chin, or you can think of dropping the elbow under the chin or pointing your wrist to the back hip
3) Rotate the upper body (squaring yourself) to the side wall at the beginning of the swing
4) Step into the shot
5) Follow through the ball using the upper body rotation whilst utilising balance in the lunge to control the shot.

Full Name: _____

Date: _____

6.3 **Q&A Task:** In your own words, write down all the steps of Handshake or V Shape grip to test your understanding? Also, define why the statement below is true?

"The squash racket grip is one of the most basic, important, and neglected parts of a squash technique whether it's on the forehand (FH) or backhand (BH)."

_____

_____

_____

_____

_____

_____

_____

_____

_____

_____

_____

_____

Full Name: _____

Date: _____

6.4 **Q&A Task:** In your own words, define why the statement below is true and write down all the steps of the three stages of the technique?

"Preparation of the racket from the "T" is one of the most crucial and important parts in striking a clean ball. Without solid preparation, one cannot move and strike a clean ball because one won't have the time due to the racket not being prepared and in the right position."

_____

_____

_____

_____

_____

_____

_____

_____

_____

_____

_____

Full Name: _____

Date: _____

6.5   Q&A Task: In your own words, write down all the steps of the forehand (FH) technique?

_____

_____

_____

_____

_____

_____

_____

_____

_____

_____

_____

_____

_____

_____

_____

_____

Full Name: _____

Date: _____

6.6 **Q&A Task:** In your own words, write down all the steps of the backhand (BH) technique?

_____

_____

_____

_____

_____

_____

_____

_____

_____

_____

_____

_____

_____

_____

_____

Section Seven

Court Movement

7.1 Fundamentals of Movement

Moving smoothly and efficiently on the squash court is one of the most significant factors that play a big part in differentiating between different levels. One of the things often not realised when it comes to the squash movement is the difference between being 'early' on the ball and 'rushing'. If one moves recklessly and rushes to the ball by moving fast and taking lots of unnecessary lunges, then one is bound to play a very loose shot because the movement is rushed and not controlled to the ball. On the contrary, if one move early and controls the ball then one can get on the ball with an appropriate amount of speed without taking unnecessary lunges which results in one hitting tight shots and shots into the targeted areas. In addition, there must be a balance when it comes to moving correctly on a squash court.

The speed and pace of movement on a squash court should change as needed. Moving too fast with no control will impact shot quality, and moving too slow will make it hard to retrieve certain shots. It's best to maintain a balanced position and take the appropriate amount of lunges, whether attacking or defending.

Movement in the 4 Quadrants:

When looking to move on a squash court, there are six basic areas of the court which must be practised when learning the fundamentals of court movement. The first part of the movement covers the two front parts of the court or, as stated earlier, Quadrants 1 and 2. Quadrant 1 is the front left part of the court, and Quadrant 2 is the front-right part of the court. Generally, one plays backhand shots from Quadrants 1 and 3 and forehand shots from Quadrants 2 and 4. ***(Refer to Illustration 43: Quadrant 1 Movement – Front BH, Illustration 44: Quadrant 2 Movement – Front FH, Illustration 45: Short or Front-Line Movement - Mid BH, Illustration 46: Short or Front-Line Movement - Mid FH, Illustration 47: Quadrant 3: Movement – Back BH and Illustration 48: Quadrant 4: Movement – Back FH)***

To move correctly in the front corners, one must take a neutral stance on the "T" and, when committed to move to the front backhand or forehand corner. One must then take strides or lunges. It is vital to always move straight to the ball, which means taking the direct path to the ball or the inside line. At the start, it is best to always end up on one's front leg or traditional leg. On the front backhand corner, the traditional or front leg is the right leg and on the front forehand corner, the traditional or front leg is the left leg. When one is finished with the shot, then one can move out of the shot in an arc to get back to the "T". The movement pattern is identical to a leaf shape. It is absolutely vital for one to use the momentum of the shot to get back to the "T" and not stop and start once the shot is played because one loses momentum.

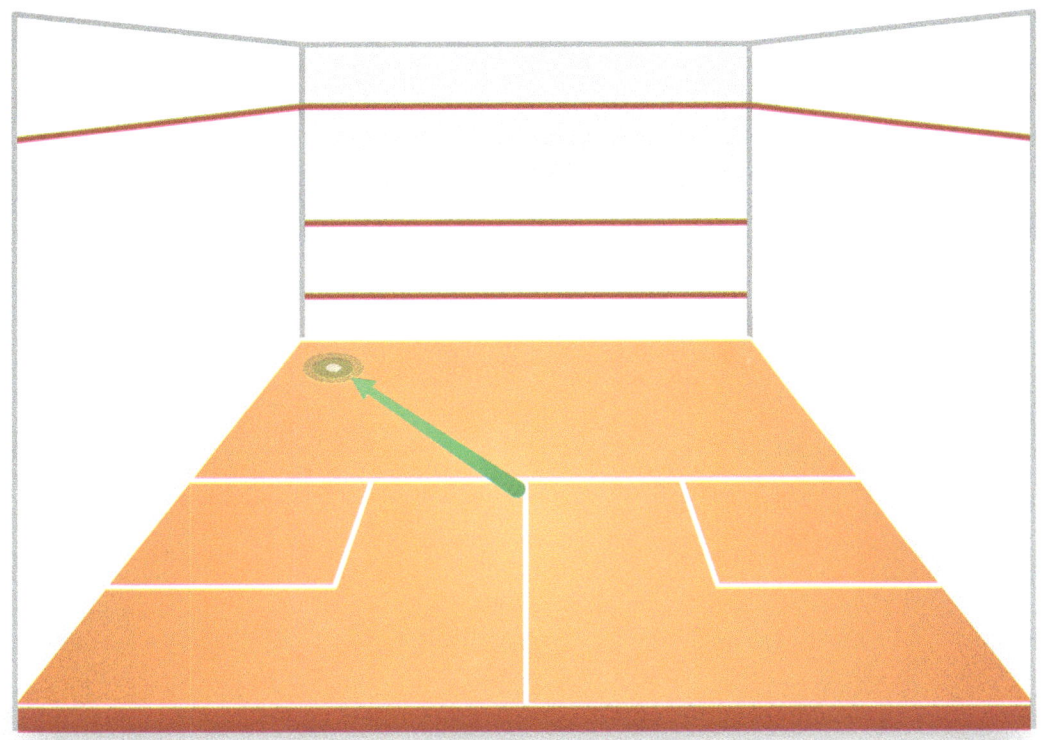

Illustration 43: Quadrant 1 Movement – Front BH

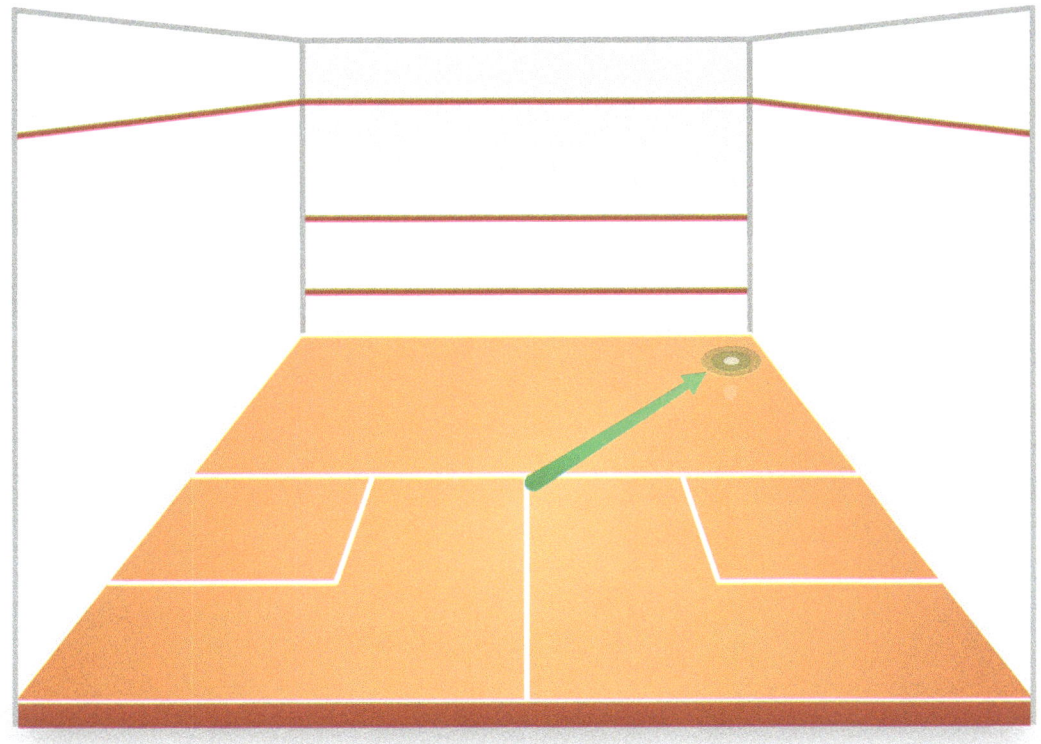

Illustration 44: Quadrant 2 Movement – Front FH

Next, we cover the middle part of the court around the short or front-line area. This is one of the most important parts of the court because this is where one is on the "T" and looks to volley or cut an opponent's shot to take the time away. To move correctly on the front or short line, one must take a neutral stance on the "T" and when committed to moving either on the forehand or backhand. You can practice moving forward by taking strides at an angle to cut the ball in front of the short or front line. In addition, one can also practice shuffle movements to cut the ball around the front or short line. The movement pattern is identical to a leaf shape.

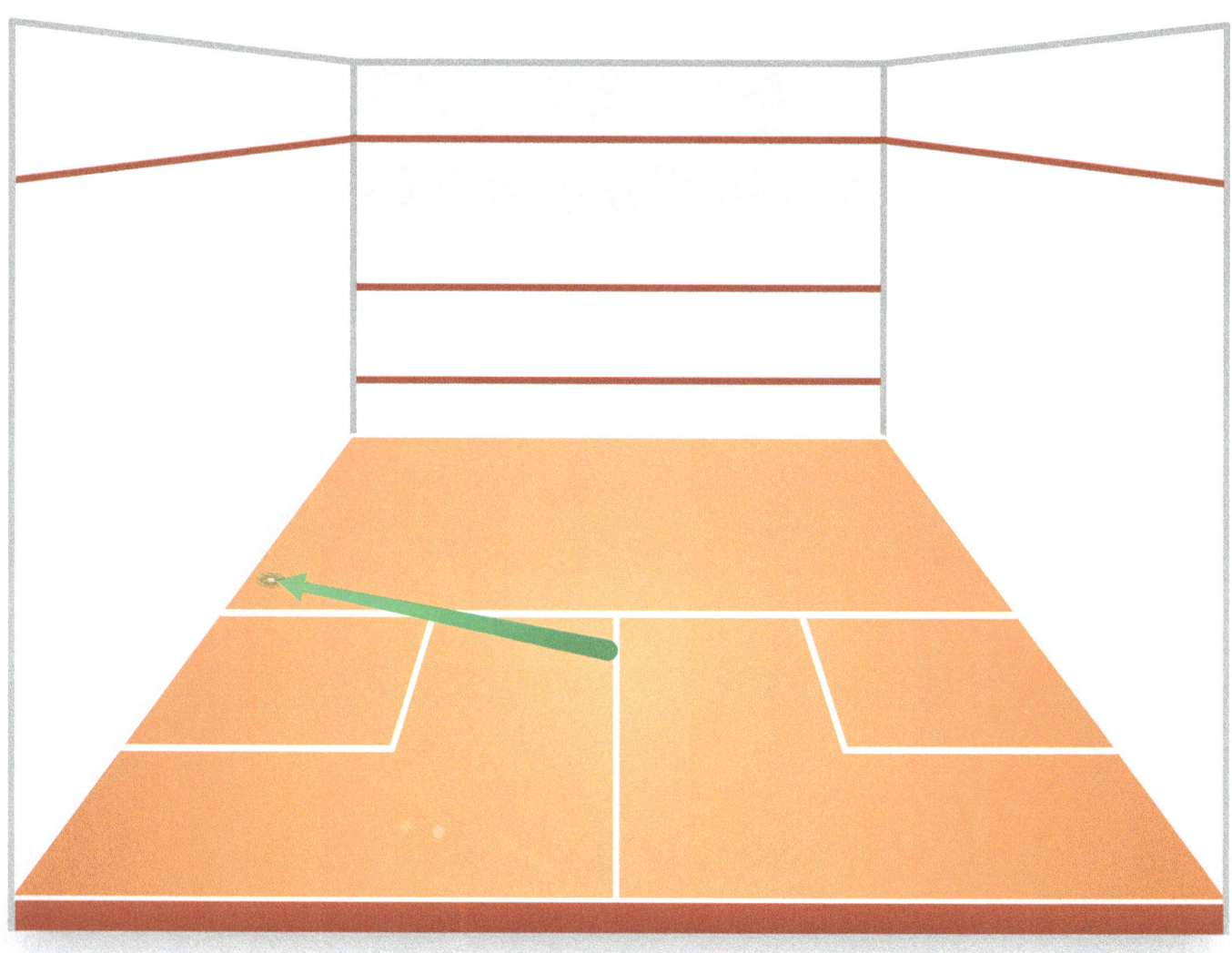

Illustration 45: Short or Front-Line Movement - Mid BH

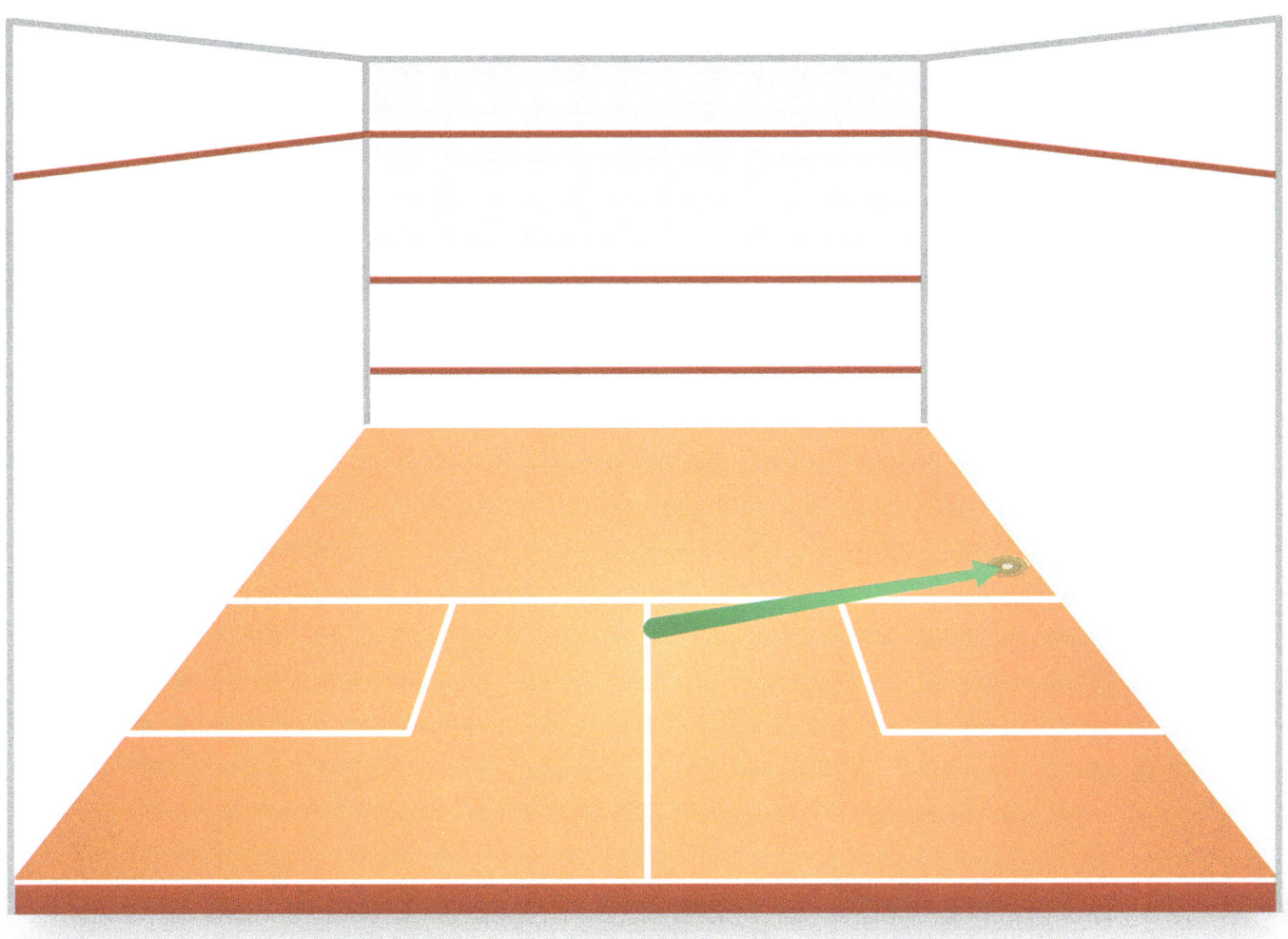

Illustration 46: Short or Front-Line Movement - Mid FH

Lastly, the back corners are where most of the game is usually played. To move in the back corners, you need to look for the volley first. If you judge that it is difficult to volley the shot, then you must take the straight or direct path to the ball to the back corner. Once the shot is hit, you can then move out of the shot in an arc and back to the "T". The movement pattern is identical to a leaf shape. The movement in the back corners are the same except one is on the backhand and one is on the forehand covering Quadrant 3 and 4. There are about five different ways to move to the back corners. For this course, we are only covering the fundamentals, but essentially, there are different variations of movements and paces in which one can practice.

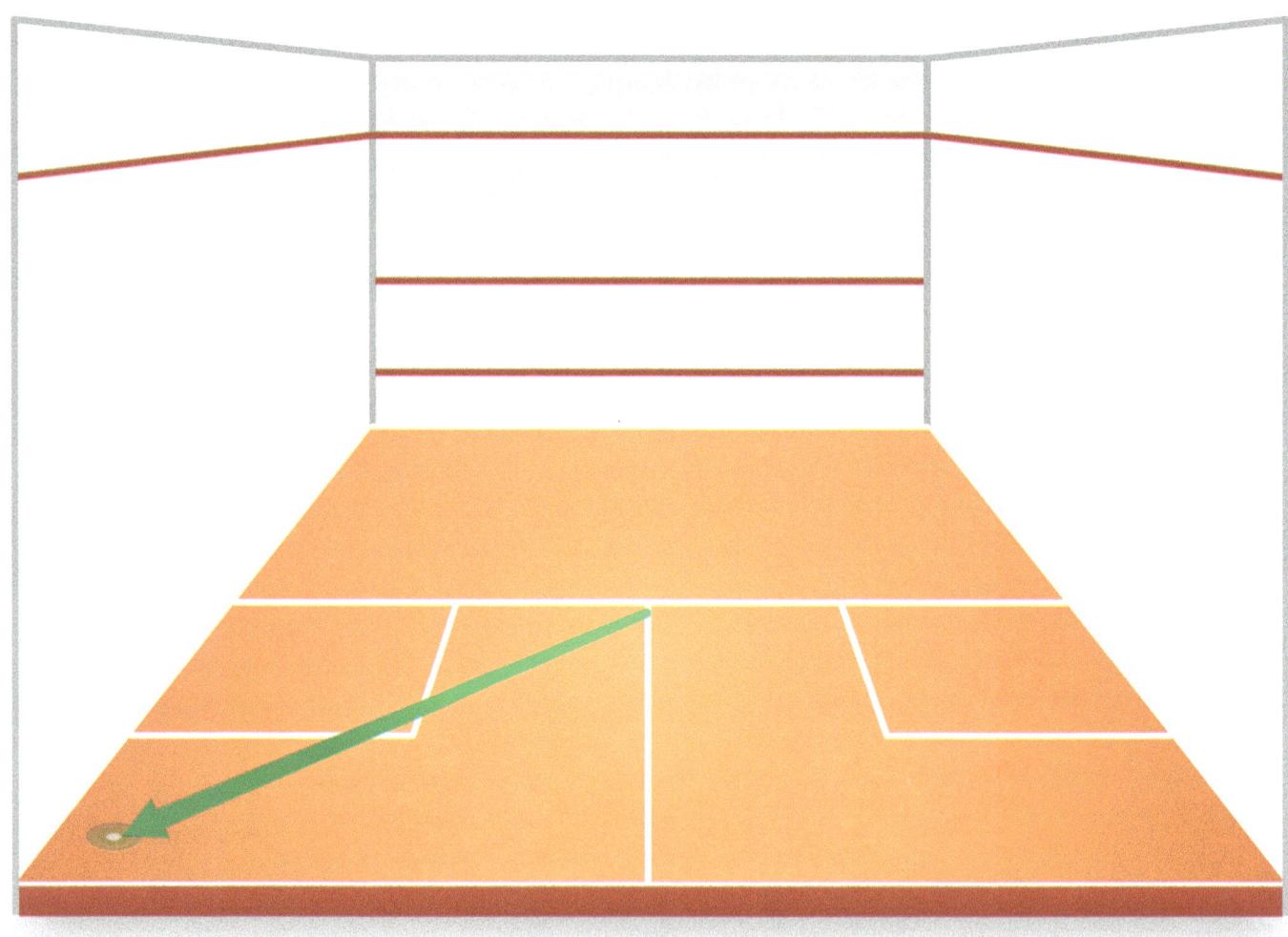

Illustration 47: Quadrant 3: Movement – Back BH

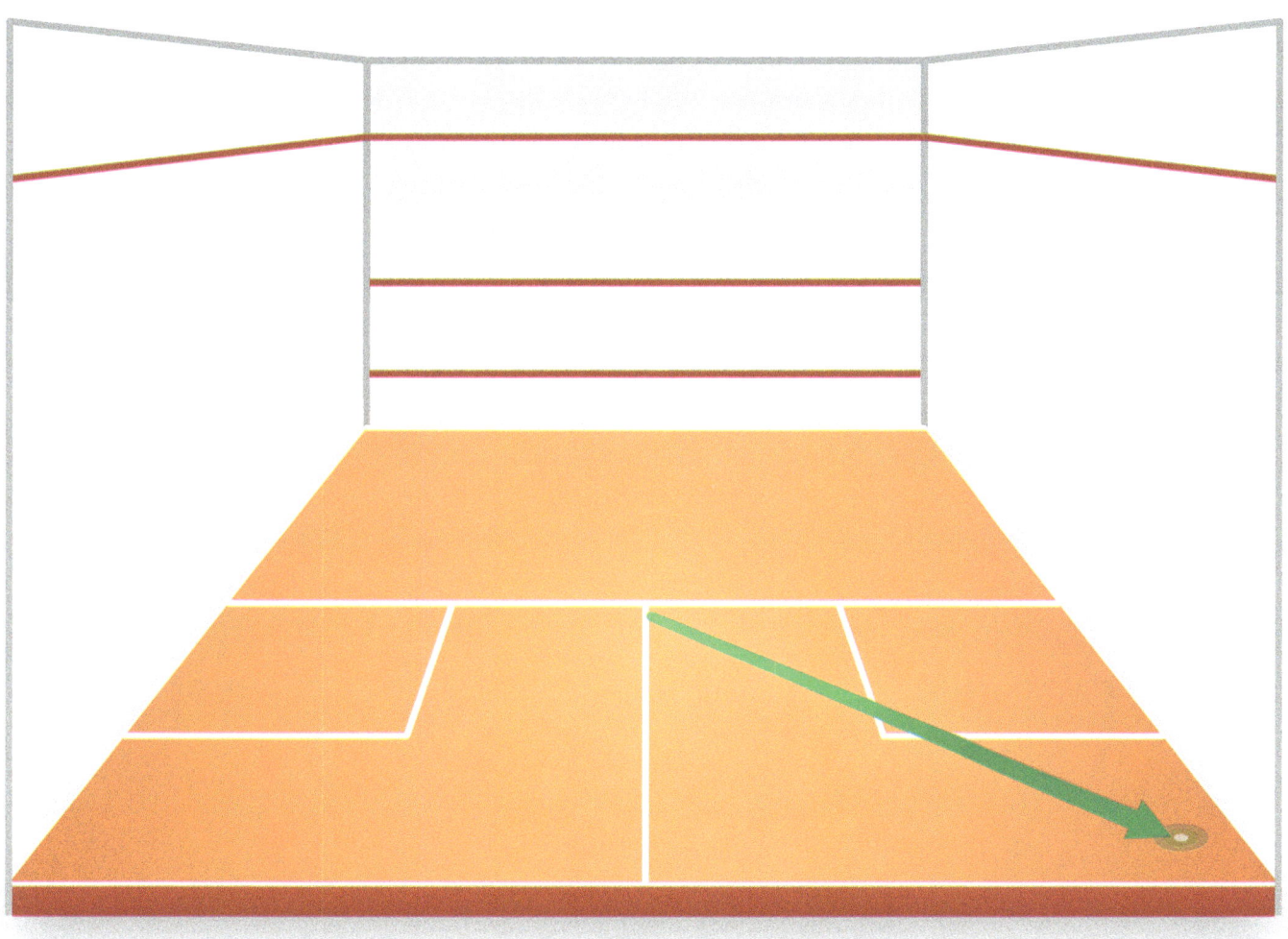

Illustration 48: Quadrant 4: Movement – Back FH

Additionally, one must focus on the timing of the movement because it is pivotal to ensure the greatest outcome when striking the ball. Timing the movement correctly also fortifies one's stability and great positioning at the point of contact which results in hitting quality shots.

In summary, movement in all corners of the court is all about momentum, balance, and timing. Momentum, balance, and timing are crucial because they each play a major role in one being early or rushed to the ball and the quality of shot played.

To get further clarity and understanding, it is best to read each movement section together with the diagram provided and most importantly apply it. Refer to the diagrams which show the path of the movement to the ball in the six basic parts of the court.

Ghosting:

Ghosting, invented by Jonah Barrington, is a valuable tool for practising movement in squash. It provides many benefits such as enhancing technique, movement, visualisation, and fitness, all without the need for a ball or a trainer. Ghosting can be done in two forms: Technical ghosting and Fitness ghosting.

Technical ghosting focuses on improving the movement patterns and technique of racket preparation, swing, lunges, and movement to the corners. It is best to practice it slowly and with control, as the goal is to learn the correct technical movement on the court.

Fitness ghosting, on the other hand, is about practicing under pressure and improving speed, endurance, and overall fitness. It is recommended to start with technical ghosting to establish a solid understanding of movement and swing before moving on to fitness ghosting.

Basic Terms:

In the following three sections, there are movement drills designed to apply the fundamentals of court movement. Before starting the movement drills, here are some terms which need to be understood. In addition, after each drill is completed, there is a Q&A sheet which must be completed to discuss one's success and the results (or sequel) achieved after the movements drills are completed. The movement drills can be done by an individual by themself, with a training partner or a coach.

Name:

Name can be defined as a word or set of words by which a person or thing is to be addressed or referred to as, in this case, the way a drill is going to be referred to.

Target:

Target is an objective or results towards which efforts are directed.

Drill:

Drill provides instructions and steps for a particular drill to be performed.

End Sequel:

End sequel or end result is meant here as one acquiring a new skill, improvement, understanding and increased ability to perform a particular drill.

MTR:

MTR is an abbreviation or short form of Movement Training Drill.

7.2 Practical: MTR-01 (Movement Training Drill-01)

Name: MTR-01, Front Court Movements

Target: To acquire the skill of being able to move to the two front parts of the court efficiently.

Drill: Front Backhand Corner: Quadrant 1

1) Place a marker on the front left-hand part of the court, typically 4 floorboards away from the side wall (horizontally) and 1.5 racket length from the tin (vertically) to create an alley
2) Start with a neutral stance on the "T" meaning (one is on their toes on the "T" with body facing the front wall, knees slightly bent and forward with racket up in front pointing on the front wall)
3) Before moving, take the racket back and up
4) Take a quick split step and move in a direct/straight path or taking the inside line to the ball
5) Lead with your left leg, followed by the right leg, left leg and ending up on the right leg which is the traditional leg
6) Play the imaginary ball by swinging through it
7) Move out of the ball taking the outside line or in an arc back to the "T"
8) The movement pattern should look like a leaf shape. *(Refer to Illustration 43: Quadrant 1 Movement – Front BH)*

Front Forehand Corner: Quadrant 2

1) Place another marker on the front right-hand part of the court, typically 4 floorboards away from the side wall (horizontally) and 1.5 racket length from the tin (vertically) to create an alley
2) Start with a neutral stance on the "T" meaning (one is on their toes on the "T" with body facing the front wall, knees slightly bent and forward with racket up in front pointing on the front wall)
3) Before moving, take the racket back and up
4) Take a quick split step and move in a direct/straight path or taking the inside line to the ball
5) Lead with your right leg, left leg, right leg and ending up on the left leg which is the traditional leg
6) Play the imaginary ball by swinging through it
7) Move out of the ball taking the outside line or in an arc back to the "T"
8) The movement pattern should look like a leaf shape. *(Refer to Illustration 44: Quadrant 2 Movement – Front FH)*

End Sequel:

When one has reached a point where one feels comfortable, efficient, and confident moving to the front parts of the court and can successfully apply the drills with hitting physical ball and in games.

Full Name: _____

Date: _____

7.3   Q&A Task: Describe any wins or results that you have gained from applying the MTR-01?

_____

_____

_____

_____

_____

_____

_____

_____

_____

_____

_____

_____

_____

_____

7.4 Practical: MTR-02 (Movement Training Drill)

Name: MTR-02, Short- line or Front- line Court Movements

Target: To acquire the skill of being able to move efficiently along the short or front line of the court and gaining control of the "T".

Drill: Short line Backhand: Volleys

1) Place a marker on the front left-hand part of the short line typically 4 floorboards away from the side wall (horizontally) and 1 meter from the short line (vertically) to create an alley
2) Start with neutral stance on the "T" meaning (one is on their toes on the "T" with body facing the front wall, knees slightly bent and forward with racket up in front pointing on the front wall)
3) Before moving, take the racket back and up
4) Take quick split step and move in an angle taking direct/straight path to the ball
5) Lead with your left leg and ending up on the right leg which is the traditional leg
6) Play the imaginary ball by swinging through it
7) Move out of the ball taking the outside line or in an arc back to the "T"
8) The movement should look like a leaf shape.*(Refer to Illustration 45: Short or Front-Line Movement - Mid BH)*

Short line Forehand: Volleys

1) Place a marker on the front right-hand part of the short line typically 4 floorboards away from the side wall (horizontally) and 1 meter from the short line (vertically) to create an alley
2) Start with a neutral stance on the "T" meaning (one is on their toes on the "T" with body facing the front wall, knees slightly bent and forward with racket up in front pointing on the front wall)
3) Before moving, take the racket back and up
4) Take a quick split step and move in an angle taking direct/straight path to the ball
5) Lead with your right leg and ending up on the left leg which is the traditional leg
6) Play the imaginary ball by swinging through it
7) Move out of the ball taking the outside line or in an arc back to the "T"
8) The movement should look like a leaf shape.*(Refer to Illustration 46: Short or Front-Line Movement - Mid FH)*

End Sequel:

One is confident moving along the short line or front line of the court and can successfully apply the movement in the drills with hitting physical balls and in games.

Full Name: _____

Date: _____

7.5 Q&A Task: Describe any wins or results that you have gained from applying the MTR-02?

_____

_____

_____

_____

_____

_____

_____

_____

_____

_____

_____

_____

_____

_____

_____

_____

_____

7.6 Practical: MTR-03 (Movement Training Drill)

Name: MTR-03, Back Court Movements

Target: To acquire the skill of efficiently moving to the two back parts of the court.

Drill: Back Backhand Corner: Quadrant 3

1) Place a marker on the back left-hand part of the court, typically 4 floorboards away from the side wall (horizontally) and 1 racket length from the back wall (vertically) to create an alley
2) Start with a neutral stance on the "T" meaning (one is on their toes on the "T" with body facing the front wall, knees slightly bent and forward with racket up in front pointing on the front wall)
3) Before moving, take the racket back and up
4) Take a quick split step, turn, and move in a direct/straight path or taking the inside line to the ball
5) Lead with your right leg, followed by the left leg and ending up on the right leg which is the traditional leg
6) Play the imaginary ball by swinging through it
7) Move out of the ball taking the outside line or in an arc back to the "T"
8) The movement should look like a leaf shape. *(Refer to Illustration 47: Quadrant 3: Movement – Back BH)*

Back Forehand Corner: Quadrant 4

1) Place another marker on the back right-hand part of the court, typically 4 floorboards away from the side wall (horizontally) and 1 racket length from the tin (vertically), to create an alley
2) Start with a neutral stance on the "T" meaning (one is on their toes on the "T" with body facing the front wall, knees slightly bent and forward with racket up in front pointing on the front wall)
3) Before moving, take the racket back and up
4) Take a quick split step, turn, and move in a direct/straight path or taking the inside line to the ball
5) Lead with your left leg, followed by the right leg and ending up on the left leg which is the traditional leg
6) Play the imaginary ball by swinging through it
7) Move out of the ball taking the outside line or in an arc back to the "T"
8) The movement should look like a leaf shape. *(Refer to Illustration 48: Quadrant 4: Movement – Back FH)*

End Sequel:

When one has reached a point where one feels efficient and confident moving in and out of the back parts of the court and can successfully apply the drills with hitting the physical ball and in games.

Full Name: _____

Date: _____

7.7 Q&A Task: Describe any wins or results that you have gained from applying the MTR-03?

_____

_____

_____

_____

_____

_____

_____

_____

_____

_____

_____

_____

_____

_____

Section Eight

Solo Training

8.1 Introduction to Solo Training

Squash is such a unique sport that it gives one the ability to practice alone, also known as Solo practice, and with others. Solo practice is one of the key elements for different levels of squash players to improve their technique, accuracy, and consistency of shots. The solo practice also develops habits and muscle memory due to repetitively hitting the shots in a particular part of the court. It is a time when one gets on the court by themselves and works on specific areas of technique, movement, and shots because it helps one analyse and break down the areas that require improvement. Some of the top and best squash players apply Solo practice to their training routine every week because it is essential to their growth.

In this course, we will discuss and cover the six basic Solo practices, which are the fundamentals of Solo training.

Backhand and Forehand Straight Drives or Length:

The BH and FH straight drives are basic yet very important shots that need your attention in a solo practice. BH and FH drives are essentially the base of the game and where most of the game is played. To practice FH drives, one starts on the Quadrant 4 on the right side of the back court. One then looks to strike the ball towards the front wall aiming at Quarter 3 and getting the ball to bounce inside Zone 2 and 3. It is also prudent to set a target of how many floorboards within a ball should bounce. One can start with 4 floorboards, and as one improves and gets confident, one can go to 3, 2 and 1 floorboards. The idea is to have good racket preparation, good footwork, tracking of the ball and hitting straight drives repeatedly as tight to the sidewall as possible on the first bounce. Practising BH drives is the same as the FH drives, but it's on the Quadrant 3 on the left side of the back court.

Backhand and Forehand Straight Volleys:

Volleying is another important attacking shot for solo practice. To practice volley FH drives, one stands on the short line on the right side of the court and hits the ball down the line, aiming at Quarter 3. The idea is to hit the volleys repetitively and as many times as possible. Racket preparation, quick footwork and tracking the ball is essential. When practising repetitive volleys, one must be light on feet, which means staying on toes so it can help with getting in good positions to volley the next shot. The same principles apply to the volley BH drives, but one stands on the left side of the court.

Backhand and Forehand Straight Drops:

Practicing FH and BH drop shots are vital to one's game. When doing Solo practice, one needs to practice FH and BH drops to the front of the court. One can start on the "T" along the short line and feed oneself a high shot, and then follow up with a short shot, nice and soft, to the front FH corner in Quadrant 2. The aim is to keep the ball as short as possible at the front without hitting the "T". To play effective drop shots, one looks to aim at Quarter 1 on the front wall with the aim of either playing a tight drop shot glued on the side wall or playing a drop so it nicks in the corner. It is also prudent to set a target of how many floorboards within a ball should bounce. One can start with 4 floorboards, and as one improves and gets confident, one can then go to 3, 2 and 1 floorboard. The basis of drop shots is the same on the BH side, except one is looking to put the ball inside Quadrant 1 as short as possible on the front part of the court without making an error or hitting the tin.

Summary:

While Solo practice is important for one's growth, it is equally important to keep the session of high quality. It is best to always train quality over quantity. When doing Solo practice, keep your session to maximum 30 minutes to keep up with the quality and improvement.

8.2 Practical: STR-01 (Solo Training Drill)

Name: STR-01, Forehand Drives, Backhand Drops and Forehand Volleys

Target: To acquire the skill of being able to hit FH straight drives repetitively from the back of the court (Quadrant 4), BH drop shots from the front of the court (Quadrant 1) within 4 floorboards and repetitive FH volley drives around the short or front line.

Drill: Forehand Drives: Back Corner (Quadrant 4)

1) Place a marker on the back right-hand part of the court typically 4 floorboards away from the side wall (horizontally) and 1.5 racket length from the back wall (vertically) to create an alley
2) Set a timer for a total of 5 minutes
3) Start the timer and take your position between Zone 2 and 3 in Quadrant 4
4) Start by hitting straight drives on the first bounce by aiming on Quarter 3 (attacking drives) and Quarter 4 (defensive drives) on the front wall with the aim of getting the ball bouncing inside Zone 2 or 3 in the back corner
5) Key technical elements important to remember for this drill are:
    - Racket up and back
    - Quick footwork to ensure that body is always behind the ball or ball in front of you when striking
    - Body rotation and transfer of weight into the shot
    - Follow through the ball

Backhand Drop shots: Front left-hand Corner (Quadrant 1)

1) Place a marker on the front left-hand part of the court typically 4 floorboards away from the side wall (horizontally) and 1 racket length from the back wall (vertically) to create an alley
2) Set a timer for a total of 5 minutes
3) Start the timer and take your position on the "T"
4) Feed ball to yourself inside Quadrant 1 at around Quarter 1 or 2 on the front wall
5) Start by hitting straight BH drop shots on the first bounce by aiming on Quarter 1 (attacking drops) on the front wall with the aim of getting the ball as tight to the side wall as possible
6) Make sure to mix up your feeding so you are always looking to get in good positions and playing BH drop shots from different parts of Quadrant 1
7) Key technical elements important to remember for this drill are:
    - Racket up and back after you feed the ball
    - Quick footwork to ensure that body is always behind the ball or ball in front of you when playing the drop shot
    - Body rotation and transfer of weight into the shot
    - Follow through the ball and softening up the hands
    - Ball must be played nice, soft, and tight along the side wall.

Drill: Forehand Repetitive Volleys: Short or Front line

1) Set a timer for a total of 5 minutes
2) Start the timer and take your position on the short or front line on the right-hand side of the court about 1 to 1.5 racket away from the sidewall
3) Start by hitting straight volley drives without any bounce repetitively by aiming on Quarter 3 on the front wall
4) Key technical elements important to remember for this drill are:
   - Racket up and back
   - Track the ball as the ball will come back fast
   - Quick footwork to ensure that body is always behind the ball or ball in front of you when striking
   - Body rotation and transfer of weight into the shot
   - Follow through the ball

End Sequel:

When one has reached a point where one can hit consistently, FH drives to the back corner, BH drops shots into the front left-hand corner and repetitive FH volleys from the short or front line.

Full Name: _____

Date: _____

8.3 Q&A Task: Describe any wins or results you have gained from applying the STR-01?

_____

_____

_____

_____

_____

_____

_____

_____

_____

_____

_____

_____

_____

_____

_____

8.4 Practical: STR-02 (Solo Training Drill)

Name: STR-02, Backhand Drives, Forehand Drops and Backhand Volley

Target: To acquire the skill of being able to hit BH straight drives repetitively from the back of the court (Quadrant 4), FH drop shots from the front of the court (Quadrant 2) within 4 floorboards and repetitive BH volley drives around the short or front line

Drill: Backhand Drives: Back Corner (Quadrant 3)

1) Place a marker on the back left-hand part of the court typically 4 floorboards away from the side wall (horizontally) and 1.5 racket length from the back wall (vertically) to create an alley
2) Set a timer for a total of 5 minutes
3) Start the timer and take your position between Zone 2 and 3 in Quadrant 3
4) Start by hitting straight drives on the first bounce by aiming on Quarter 3 (attacking drives) and Quarter 4 (defensive drives) on the front wall with the aim of getting the ball bouncing inside Zone 2 or 3 in the back corner
5) Key technical elements important to remember for this drill are:
   - Racket up and back
   - Quick footwork to ensure that body is always behind the ball or ball in front of you when striking
   - Body rotation and transfer

Forehand Drop shots: Front right-hand Corner (Quadrant 2)

1) Place a marker on the front right-hand part of the court typically 4 floorboards away from the side wall (horizontally) and 1 racket length from the back wall (vertically) to create an alley
2) Set a timer for a total of 5 minutes
3) Start the timer and take your position on the "T"
4) Feed ball to yourself inside Quadrant 2 at around Quarter 1 or 2 on the front wall
5) Start by hitting straight FH drop shots on the first bounce by aiming on Quarter 1 (attacking drops) on the front wall with the aim of getting the ball as tight to the side wall as possible
6) Make sure to mix up your feeding so you are always looking to get in good positions and playing FH drop shots from different parts of Quadrant 2
7) Key technical elements important to remember for this drill are:
   - Racket up and back after you feed the ball
   - Quick footwork to ensure that body is always behind the ball or ball in front of you when playing the drop shot
   - Body rotation and transfer of weight into the shot
   - Follow through the ball and softening up the hands
   - Ball must be played nice, soft, and tight along the side wall

Drill: Backhand Repetitive Volleys: Short or Front line

1) Set a timer for a total of 5 minutes
2) Start the timer and take your position on the short or front line on the left-hand side of the court about 1 to 1.5 racket away from the sidewall
3) Start by hitting straight volley drives without any bounce repetitively by aiming on Quarter 3 on the front wall
4) Key technical elements important to remember for this drill are:
   - Racket up and back
   - Track the ball as the ball will come back fast
   - Quick footwork to ensure that body is always behind the ball or ball in front of you when striking
   - Body rotation and transfer of weight into the shot
   - Follow through the ball

End Sequel:

When one has reached a point where one can hit consistently, BH drives to the back corner, FH drop shots into the front right-hand corner and repetitive BH volley drives from the short or front line.

Full Name: _____

Date: _____

8.5 **Q&A Task:** Describe any wins or results you have gained from applying the STR-02?

_____
_____
_____
_____
_____
_____
_____
_____
_____
_____
_____
_____
_____
_____

Section Nine

Dyads Training

9.1 Introduction to Dyads Training

Dyads training, also known as pairs training consist of two players training together at a specific activity, a squash drill(s). Dyads training can be vital and has numerous benefits because it not only helps one player to improve but also, the twin. The drills can be run so that the twins can focus on a particular shot or movement. It also makes it fun for both twins. Dyads drills can be structured to simulate the squash game or even a particular rally pattern. There are several drill activities that dyads can practice together. It is important that whilst doing dyads training, the twins focus on:

- Setting the target for the session
- Amount of drills to be drilled
- Duration of the session
- Focus of each twin and the shots or movement to be drilled

It is essential to have a set target whether it is Solo training, Dyads training or Match plays. Without a target, the session can lose its quality, and the twin's focus can be lost. An example of a good, planned session can be:

- Target is to improve straight drives to the back corners
- There will be two types of drills that will be performed
- Duration of the session is 40 minutes in total
- Twin A is focusing on early racket preparation, and Twin B is focusing on body position.

Structuring the session like the above can make the entire session quality and also utilise the time wisely.

9.2 Practical: DTR-01 (Dyads Training Drill)

Name: DTR-01, Three Quadrants Feeding and Striking

Target Twin A: To acquire the skill of being able to feed straight drops, straight drives and boasts consistently in sequence.

Target Twin B: To build the skill of hitting straight drives, straight volleys and crosscourt drives consistently at the targeted areas.

Drill: Straight Drop – Straight Drive, Straight Drive – Volley Straight Drive and Boast – Crosscourt Drive

To perform this drill at the best level possible, we will assign a hat to both the Twins. Twin A is the coach, and Twin B is the student. The reason for this is that one takes the role of feeding whilst the other takes the role of practising different drives. It is prudent that both Twins switch positions so that they can both practice and wear the hats of coach and student. In addition, discuss the areas you can both improve on whilst practising, as communication is the key when doing Dyads drills.

To execute this drill, follow the steps below:

1) Twin A feeds a straight drop, straight drive, and a boast in this sequence one at a time for 10 mins. The drill is done in a sequence where Twin A is the coach and Twin B is the student.
2) Twin A takes his position inside Quadrant 4 or on the forehand back corner and feeds a straight drop aiming between Quarters 1 and 2. Twin B takes his position on the 'T', and after the drop is fed, Twin B looks to hit a straight drive to the back, aiming at Quarter 2 on the front wall.
3) Twin A then feeds a straight drive by aiming between Quarter 3 and 4 on the front wall, and Twin B hits a straight volley drive to the back, aiming for Quarter 3 on the front wall.
4) Twin A feeds a two-wall or three-wall boast aiming for Quarter 1 or 2, and Twin B hits a crosscourt drive to the back corner inside Quadrant 4.
5) After the 10 mins are over, switch sides i.e., Twin A feeds from Quadrant 3 and repeats the 10 mins cycle.
6) Once the 10 mins cycle is complete for both quadrants of the court, totalling 20 mins, the Twins switch hats and positions i.e., Twin A is the student and Twin B is the coach, then continue the above steps from 1 to 5.

End Sequel:

To reach a point where both the Twins can wear the hats of coach and student and to be able to feed and hit quality shots in the targeted areas.

Full Name: _____

Date: _____

9.3 **Q&A Task:** Describe any wins or results you have gained from applying the DTR-01?

_____

_____

_____

_____

_____

_____

_____

_____

_____

_____

_____

_____

_____

_____

_____

9.4 Practical: DTR-02 (Dyads Training Drill)

Name: DTR-02, The Diagonals

Target: To acquire the skill of being able to hit boasts, cross court lobs and straight drives and practising the continuity of the drill in sequence.

Drill: Boast, Cross Lob, Straight Drive and Alternate

This is one of the best drills that can help one improve their court movement diagonally and also placement of the shots in the two opposite quadrants i.e., Quadrant 1 to 4 or Quadrant 2 to 3. In addition, discuss the areas you can improve on whilst practising, as communication is the key when doing Dyads drills.

To execute this drill, follow the below sequence:

1) Set a timer for 10 mins in total
2) Twin A starts with a boast inside Quadrant 4
3) Twin B plays a cross lob of the boast from inside Quadrant 1
4) Twin A plays a straight drive or straight volley of the lob from Quadrant 4
5) Twin B plays a boast from Quadrant 4
6) Twin A plays a cross lob of the boast from inside Quadrant 1
7) Twin B plays a straight drive or straight volley of the lob from Quadrant 4
8) The cycle of the drill continues in that sequence until both the Twins are satisfied with the drill.

Once the Twins are satisfied, then the sides must be switched, and the below sequence must be followed:

1) Set a timer again for 10 mins in total
2) Twin A starts with a boast inside Quadrant 3
3) Twin B plays a cross lob of the boast from inside Quadrant 2
4) Twin A plays a straight drive or straight volley of the lob from Quadrant 3
5) Twin B plays a boast from Quadrant 3
6) Twin A plays a cross lob of the boast from inside Quadrant 2
7) Twin B plays a straight drive or straight volley of the lob from Quadrant 3
8) The cycle continues in that sequence until both the Twins are satisfied with the drill.

End Sequel:

To reach a point where both the Twins can keep the drill continuous and can hit quality boasts, cross lobs and straight drives or straight volleys into the targeted areas of the court.

Full Name: _____

Date: _____

9.5 **Q&A Task:** Describe any wins or results that you have gained from applying the DTR-02?

_____

_____

_____

_____

_____

_____

_____

_____

_____

_____

_____

_____

_____

_____

_____

_____

Section Ten

Statistics- Result Tracking

10.1 What is a Statistic?

A statistic can be defined as an amount or number compared to a preceding amount or the number of the same thing. Statistics can be used for this course to measure the quantity, quality, and improvement of one's progress in squash.

Statistics are simple. They can be understood as follows:

An up statistic means that the current amount or number is more than the preceding one.

A down statistic means that the current amount or number is less than the preceding one.

A stable statistic means that the current amount or number is close or identical to the preceding without any improvement or deterioration.

One must keep track of one's results using the statistics for three months because, without it, one cannot accurately and properly track the results and progress. In addition, the result tracking using statistics allows one to analyse the data, receive feedback on performance, identify areas of strengths and weaknesses to help one take smart actions and to enforce discipline to improve in the areas.

Below are examples of an up statistic, a down statistic, and a stable statistic when it comes to tracking one's progress. *(Refer to Illustrations 49 to 51 – Up, Down and Stable Statistic)*

Up statistic:

Week	Amount
1	5
2	6
3	8
4	4
5	5
6	5
7	7
8	9
9	9.1
10	8.9
11	9.5
12	9.7

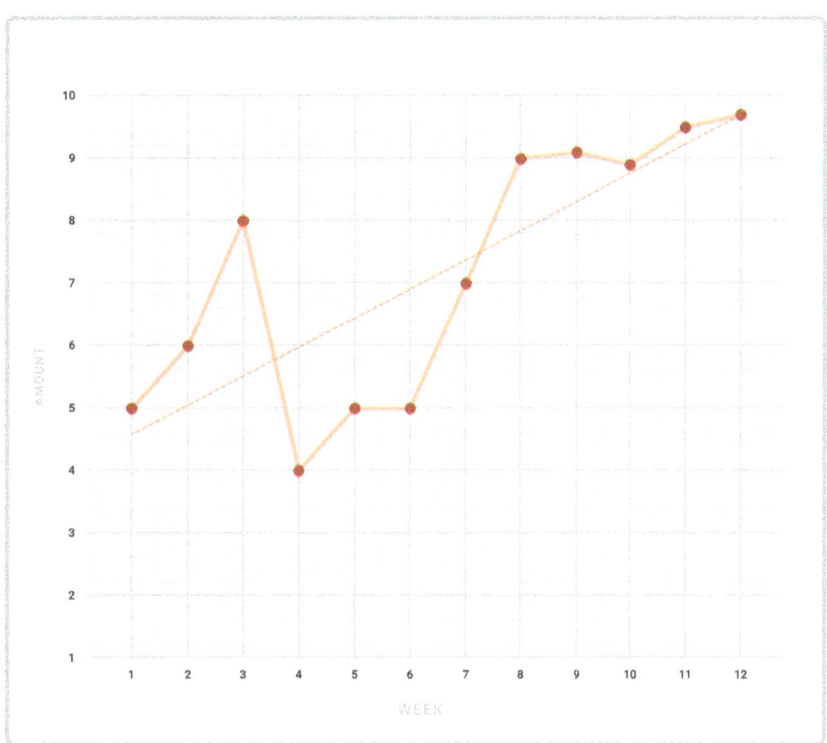

Illustrations 49: Up Statistic

Down statistic:

Week	Amount
1	9.7
2	8
3	6
4	5
5	7
6	4
7	2
8	3
9	1.5
10	2
11	4
12	1

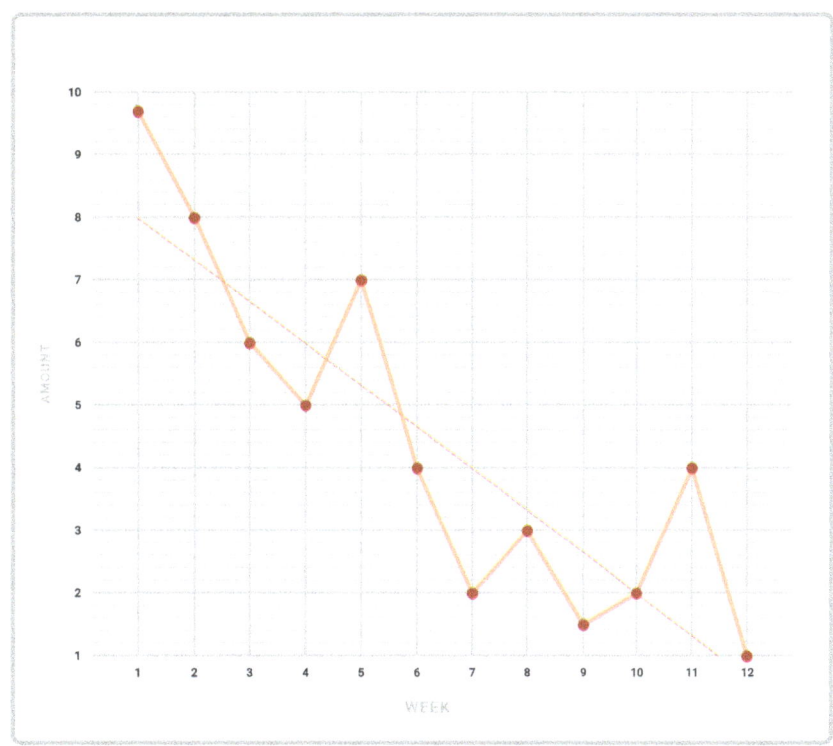

Illustrations 50: Down Statistic

Stable statistic:

Week	Amount
1	6
2	8
3	8.1
4	8.2
5	8
6	7.9
7	8.3
8	8.5
9	8.8
10	9
11	8.9
12	7

Illustrations 51: Stable Statistic

To track your progress and identify areas for improvement, use the following graph. This graph serves as a prototype to help you keep track of your progress over time. Fill in the months and year at the top of the graph to indicate the period that is being tracked. It is best to make copies of the blank graph for future use.*(Refer to Illustration 52: Blank Statistic)*

To use the graph effectively, it's important to understand the meaning of the x-axis and y-axis.

The x-axis represents a horizontal number line that displays three months broken down into twelve weeks, i.e. week 1 to week 12.

On the other hand, the y-axis displays a vertical number line that indicates the level of progress, ranging from 1 to 10, where 1 represents low progress, and 10 represents fantastic progress. Higher the number on the y-axis, better your progress. Similarly, a lower number indicates low progress.

Blank Statistic:

Week	Amount
1	
2	
3	
4	
5	
6	
7	
8	
9	
10	
11	
12	

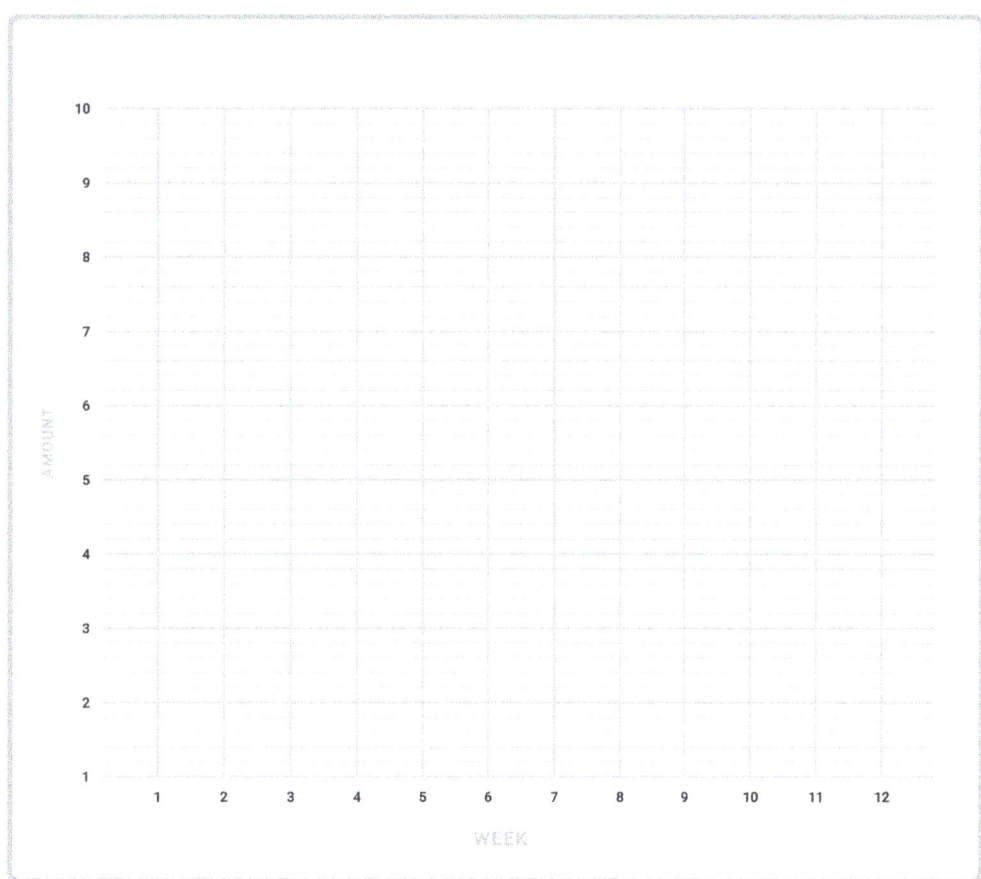

Illustrations 52: Blank Statistic

Full Name: _____

Date: _____

10.2 Q&A Task: Describe in your own words, your understanding of the below statement and draw a rough sketch of an up, down, and stable statistic?

"Statistics are simple, they can be understood as:

An up statistic means that the current amount or number is more than the preceding one.

A down statistic means that the current amount or number is less than the preceding one.

A stable statistic means that the current amount or number is close or identical to the preceding without any improvement or deterioration."

_____

_____

_____

_____

_____

_____

_____

_____

Section Eleven

Final Study Exercise

Key Takeaways

11.1 **Q&A Task:** Write about what you have learnt from this course, the key takeaways, and how can you apply the information to help you become the best squash player you can be? Go through each item below.

- a) History of Squash
- b) Squash Court
- c) Squash Court Rules
- d) Fundamentals of Technique
- e) Court Movement
- f) Solo Training Drills
- g) Dyads Training Drills
- h) Statistics- Result Tracking

_____

_____

_____

_____

_____

_____

_____

_____

Section Twelve

Appendix

Student's Accomplishment

Full Name: _____

Date: _____

12.1 Q&A Task: Write up your successes and wins from this course and how can you best apply and promote it to others?

_____

_____

_____

_____

_____

_____

_____

_____

_____

_____

www.ingramcontent.com/pod-product-compliance
Lightning Source LLC
Chambersburg PA
CBHW061134010526
44107CB00068B/2929